THE FAST LANE DIET

THE
FAST LANE
DIET

DOTTIE DEKKO

McGRAW-HILL BOOK COMPANY

New York St. Louis San Francisco Auckland Bogotá
Guatemala Hamburg Johannesburg Lisbon London
Madrid Mexico Montreal New Delhi Panama Paris
San Juan São Paulo Singapore Sydney Tokyo Toronto

1 2 3 4 5 6 7 8 9 D O C D O C 8 7 6 5

ISBN 0-07-016298-0

Library of Congress Cataloging in Publication Data
Dekko, Dottie.
The fast lane diet.
1. Reducing diets.   I. Title.
RM222.2.D45   1985   613.2′5   85-145
ISBN 0-07-016298-0

Book design by M.R.P. Design.

This book is dedicated:

To my fast-tracking 76-year-old mother, who looks as elegant in her size 5 skirt as she did 50 years ago. She is my inspiration.

And to my father, who has taught all of us about the beauty, satisfaction, and rewards of the Fast Lane.

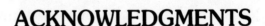

ACKNOWLEDGMENTS

Without the help and encouragement of a lot of people, this book would never have been written. I am so grateful that I have the opportunity to thank:

My husband, Tom, who has always thought that I could do anything.

My children—Danna, Lezlie, Gigi, and Jeff—who have always encouraged me to follow my ideas and have told me that I am the best mom in the world.

Two dear friends, Wendy and Jonathon Lazear, who made this whole thing happen.

My good friends Marge Heegaard, Dorothy Gores, Gail Showers, Carolyn Reichow, Bev Roeckers, and many others, all of whom have encouraged me by using my Diet Drink and losing the weight they wanted to lose.

Ann Burkhardt, a good friend and Taste Editor of *The Minneapolis Star and Tribune*, who gave me great recipes and good advice.

Arlene Stansfeld, director of consumer affairs for Land-O-Lakes, who gave me nutritional advice and encouragement.

Jeanette Lowry, M.D., my internist, who gave me her professional advice and words of encouragement.

The March of Dimes staff, who have worked with me on many projects and who have always been supportive.

Joe Mickel of Arndt & Berthiaume, the photographer who made me look my best.

Muriel Humphrey Brown, Pat Grant, and *The Minneapolis Star and Tribune*, who granted me the use of their recipes.

And Milton Seifert, Jr., M.D.

CONTENTS

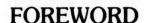

FOREWORD

It is true—nearly all of us live in the fast lane. Most of us are trying to achieve excellence in a profession, school, business, politics, sports, or homemaking. We are a country of aggressive, high-performance people. We have high expectations of ourselves. Each of us is trying to achieve a personal best.

Body weight management is an area of frequent failure, but it doesn't have to be. Like all successful endeavors, weight loss requires a mastery of fundamentals—and good nutrition is the key fundamental. When you live in the fast lane, good nutrition is even more important. Now Dottie Dekko shows us that good nutrition and weight loss do not have to be in conflict.

The Fast Lane Diet is a simple, safe, affordable, portable, and convenient diet. It is an alternative to junk food and empty calories. It does not fatigue the taste buds or your commitment to weight reduction. We have needed a guide to the leaner canned, prepared, and frozen foods. We have needed answers for coping with the business lunch, with food shopping, and with being on the road. And when our weight goal is reached, we have needed a maintenance plan. Now we have them.

Dottie Dekko raises some very important points. Dottie's recipe for the Fast Lane Diet Drink for those with lactose intolerance is very much needed. Both recipes are delicious, but they are also perfect for the millions of people in the fast lane who simply cannot have milk in their diets.

And Dottie also warns against foods high in sodium, an increasing danger with the preponderance of frozen, canned, and prepared convenience foods, in which salt and other sodium compounds are often found as preservatives.

The research that's been made available to the medical profession shows that a nondemanding diet that is easy to follow and offers tasty variety is the diet that coincides with most people's eating schedules and eating habits.

Some fast-laners will be tempted to try each diet—to mix them, or to operate on two simultaneously. Try not to. Each of the six Fast Lane Diets is designed for specific fast lane lifestyles and needs. And each one may be made less effective if you try a fast lane "composite."

Dottie Dekko helps us set reasonable weight reduction goals. She has thought about us, and she understands. This book will add to the skills with which we manage our lives.

MILTON H. SEIFERT, JR., M.D.

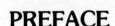

PREFACE

The world is moving at a faster and faster pace, and few of us can avoid what we call the "fast lane" of life. Probably most of us don't want to avoid it—there are countless rewards from the fast lane if we put some effort into it.

Look at your life situation this way. When everything is moving so fast that it all seems to be a blur, it is absolutely necessary that you set your priorities. Your list of priorities could include work, family, music, art, religion, or whatever, but at the top of the list *must* be care for yourself. That is what this book is about. If you don't care for yourself, none of the other priorities can be possible.

This book tells you how I learned to care for myself. Please let it help you. The Fast Lane Diet has helped countless others who live, work, and flourish in the fast lane.

DOTTIE DEKKO

THE FAST LANE DIET

HOW I CAME TO DEVELOP THE FAST LANE DIET

When I was 11 years old, I filled in for one of my father's employees at his dairy retail outlet. What started as pinch-hitting after school soon became my job all the way through to graduation from high school. At 17 I entered college, and I really found myself in a hurry. I graduated in three years rather than four and immediately embarked on my career. I taught high school students, but because I was so young, I was often taken for a student. After a year, I got restless and decided to take my diploma and my year's worth of experience and move on.

Move on I did—as home economist for one of the northern Midwest's largest utilities. All this happened a few years ago. The term "fast lane" hadn't even been invented although I was certainly in it. At this giant utility all the newly employed females had to promise not to get married for the first year on the job! Have times ever changed—thank God! The whole time that I was working during the day I was also teaching adult night school and I was superbusy.

Then Tom came into my life, and we got married. I continued working both jobs. But then my daytime employer handed

1

down another rule to us "gals." No female employee could work beyond the fifth month of pregnancy, and we could not return to our jobs until the baby was over 1 year old! Fortunately, I didn't want to.

Staying very much in the fast lane and going faster and faster came to be my pace in the next four years, during which I had three baby girls.

While our daughters were babies, Tom took a high-profile job as a corporate executive. In the new capacity of corporate wife, I had to be the entertainer, a role which I enjoy but which requires endless energy. One night Tom and I would be hosts at a cocktail party—the next night there'd be a cookout at home. Then two days later, a company picnic at the lake. All the while I was freelancing by charting 350 New York Stock Exchange over-the-counter stocks and making 20 percent on most investments (in a very soft market). I was also a full-time mom, with three daughters who kept me behind the wheel of the family car with piano lessons, ballet lessons, the swimming team (two trips across town each day for three seasons of the year), gymnastics, cheerleading practice, Campfire Girls, Girl Scouts, Brownies, guitar lessons, school choir, church choir, voice lessons, hockey practice, flute lessons, Little League baseball, dancing lessons, ice-skating lessons, ski lessons, acting lessons, and soccer lessons.

You name it. Then came the news of a fourth baby on the way. It was a boy. While Jeffrey was a baby, I was on the board of the American Association of University Women, the United Way Charities, and a whole range of school-related committees.

Then two friends and I dreamed up the ultimate in time-consuming projects. It may be hard to believe, but we started the Minnesota Kicks Soccer Team. I helped sell over 4,000 season tickets before the first season ever began. I was raising a family with four kids, working sixty to seventy hours a week in the Kicks office, and putting together my first book, *Cooking for Kicks*, when suddenly it all hit me.

It happened one day when I was driving down the highway from one meeting to the next. I was nearly 15 pounds overweight—more like 20 to 25 on the average person. I had gained the weight little by little, a few pounds after each pregnancy

2

and more while testing hundreds of recipes for the cookbook. I looked terrible and felt worse.

And then a light went on in my head: The lifestyle of a young, busy mother dictated eating on the run, eating foods high in starch and empty calories, munching between meals just to keep my energy level on the same level as my obligations. I needed a dietary aid that would allow me to keep up my day-to-day pace and not inhibit my lifestyle.

And that's when I began to develop the Fast Lane Diet Drink. Because of my background as a home economist and because I was in the middle of working on a cookbook, I already had a respectable amount of information on nutrition. What I knew about a balanced diet I applied to my own lifestyle, and soon I had a system of eating that afforded me everything I needed: delicious, totally flexible, and portable. I lost all the weight I had been gaining, and I didn't have to stop everything I was doing to count calories, weigh my meals, or study each portion of my daily food intake. What's more, my diet drink— and the handful of meals I designed to go along with it—didn't inhibit me from eating in restaurants, entertaining my husband's clients, or making separate meals for the rest of the family.

And a very important bonus: The Diet Drink never bored me—I made it in so many flavors and in so many ways that I never had a chance to "fall off" my diet. The Diet Drink never got in my way—it went right along with me. And that's the beauty of it. The Fast Lane Diet Drink and Fast Lane Diet plan go where you go, do what you do, work with *your* fast lane lifestyle.

That's why I know that the Fast Lane Diet is truly the diet for the eighties. It was developed out of necessity—the need for total flexibility, the need for high-performance nutrition, and the need to live a long, prosperous, and fit fast lane life.

2

ARE YOU IN THE
FAST LANE?

Answer true or false to each of the following statements.

At the end of the day, I find myself thinking about all the things I didn't get to accomplish.

It is sometimes difficult for me to concentrate because I am thinking three jobs ahead of the one I am currently doing.

I have found myself at the supermarket checkout with no money and no checks.

I often schedule myself for two appointments simultaneously.

I feel that other people need my time as much as or more than I do.

I find myself flipping through magazines without reading them.

I sometimes feel a desperate need to be alone.

I have run out of gas or come close to it numerous times in the past year.

My boss and loved one have accused me of getting my priorities confused.

I have sometimes been the last one to board the airplane.

I have had to miss a play or special event at my child's school.

I have let my car go months without servicing or washing because I just didn't have the time to get it done.

I have found myself making holiday decorations at the last minute—even in the middle of the night on the eve of the holiday.

I am often shocked to find out the time.

I often wonder where some of my friends have gone.

I get impatient on the road—I want the cars ahead of me to move faster.

I often finish other people's sentences for them.

People have called me a "type A" personality.

Near the end of a meal at a restaurant, I often find myself asking for the check, even before my partner is finished eating.

After a frantic morning of getting the children off to school, I sometimes find more than one half-full coffee cup around the house.

I have hailed a cab even though my bus was in plain sight.

I really resent people putting me on hold on the telephone.

I'm a terrible passenger; no one ever moves fast enough for me.

I eat some meals while standing over a sink or talking on the phone.

I have run out of excuses for being late.

If *true* is your answer to most of the above questions, believe me, you can be classified as a member in good standing of the fast lane. And the last thing you need or want is a time-consuming, crackpot diet.

What follows is a diet plan for *you*—a six-diet Fast Lane Program with an in-depth quiz that will tell you which Fast Lane Diet is made for your fast lane lifestyle.

3

WHY YOU NEED THE FAST LANE DIET

I've told you the story of how I ended up in the fast lane. Think back, and you can probably figure out how you got there, too.

When did the pace start picking up for you? In high school? In college? The day you got your first "real" job? The day you were married? The moment you reached out for your newborn child? The month before you moved into the home of your own you'd been planning and saving for?

If it's tough to pin down the precise second in time when you stomped on the gas, don't worry. It's my belief that life in the fast lane is something most of us have been living with (or trying to live with) since day one simply because the fast lane is a condition of the age we live in.

There's never been a time when things have moved as quickly as they have in the years following World War II. I'm talking about social changes, technological changes, economic changes, changes in attitudes—you name it. Change is something that not only takes getting used to; it also takes keeping up with. Most Americans are frantically trying to do just that.

You can see it in how we dress, how we look, how we behave,

how we spend our leisure moments. What's the most popular personal sport today? Running. What's the latest fashion fabric? Wash and wear cotton-polyester blend—the same stuff sweat clothes are made of. Where do many American families go for dinner on their nights out? A fast-food restaurant. Better yet, a drive-through fast-food restaurant. We practically live in our cars. We've gone from drive-in movies to drive-in banks and even drive-in churches!

Both men and women are opting for hairstyles that take little or no effort to maintain—just wash, blow-dry, and dash out the door. You don't have the patience it takes to tie your shoes? Buy some with Velcro fasteners. Can't wait for the chicken to thaw? Program the microwave!

If Aesop were writing his fables today, I'll bet he'd give the one about the tortoise and the hare an entirely different treatment. No more "slow and steady wins the race"—not in our world! Instead, the moral might be "hustle, don't look back, and above all don't stop to rest!"

Assuming that the old "survival-of-the-fittest" theory still holds true, then today's "fittest" are those who can keep pace with the changing times.

But fast-laners don't just want to keep pace. They want to get ahead. They're not satisfied with running with the pack; they aim to grab—and hold—the lead. Remember that the fast lane has always been the passing lane. Anybody who's traveling at less than maximum speed had better stay out of the way!

Fast-laners are people who won't take slow for an answer. They're on the road to success—financial, spiritual, or social (or, better yet, all three)—and they want it soon—better yet, right *now*.

Here are some fast-laners I know:

- The chairman of the board of a major corporation who gets up at 4:30 every morning to catch up on his reading
- The junior accountant struggling to get new clients
- The mother of three kids under 7 who's keeping a household together while still doing volunteer work
- The graduate student cramming for two oral exams

- The college professor rushing through the grading of sixty-five finals and then turning to the second draft of an important scholarly paper due yesterday
- The PTA president racing home to make a gourmet dinner for six
- The mother of a newborn who also has a demanding job in the garment industry

What do these people have in common? They've all set high standards for themselves—and higher goals. They know where they're going and spend much of their energy trying to get there, certain they'll make it.

What else do they have in common? Well, they've all got the qualities necessary for success—drive, ambition, energy, willpower. But they lack something people used to have plenty of before the world started speeding up and getting crazy—*time*. They barely have enough of it to meet the demands of each busy day, and they never have enough of it to spare.

They take chances, risks, and opportunities; but they seldom take care of themselves. When they opt for life in the fast lane, they abandon good eating habits. They survive on junk food because it's quick and easy, which means that they overindulge in empty calories. They're always on the move, but they hardly ever exercise.

And that's why the pounds start creeping up on them. Fast-laners often end up overweight, underexercised, and out of shape for reasons that will be explained.

As a fast lane frequenter, you probably get to most places well ahead of your peers, including the middle-age fork in the road. There's a point at which the excess fat you're carrying around stops keeping your flesh firm and rosy and starts giving in to the pull of gravity.

Middle-age weight gain hits early when one frequents the fast lane. I'm definitely there, and my 28-year-old daughter is, too. So, too, are millions of post-World War II babies—the baby-boomers.

Baby-boomers have a particularly difficult time maintaining their positions in the fast lane simply because there are so *many*

11

of them. Talk about traveling in a crowd! They're the ones who packed the colleges in the 1960s, glutted the job market in the 1970s, and are currently scrambling for footholds on the ladder to success. There are times when I'm glad I'm not in my thirties anymore. There are some *56 million* baby-boomers out there today. Being part of that group must be like running the New York Marathon—shoulder to shoulder all the way.

So why do fast-laners tend to be overweight? There are lots of reasons. Here are a few.

Your basal metabolic rate declines.

I'll explain. Generally speaking, your basal metabolic rate—or BMR—is your "idling speed." It's a measure of how many calories your body burns when you're not really doing much of anything; you might even be sleeping.

Your BMR drops as you get older, and you stop burning as many calories as you used to. The reason is probably the increase in the amount of body fat on your body. As your BMR gets lower, you need fewer calories to sustain your body. If you keep taking in the same number of calories you're accustomed to, some will turn to fat, and your BMR will drop even more. You get the picture.

Your random activity decreases as you get older. Your movements become more purposeful, and fewer calories are required to sustain your day-to-day activities.

Remember how you used to run around as a child? Climbing trees, riding your bike up and down hills, chasing your kid brother or sister? Remember how you used to squirm in your seat in school?

The older you get, the more efficient your movements become. You do what you must in fluid motions and without wasting energy. You save up tasks that require walking until you can accomplish several at once—or you delegate them to someone else.

In other words, you become sedentary.

* * *

Often you can afford to buy richer, more fattening foods.

Lobster with melted butter. Chocolate torte. Zillion-year-old Scotch. Creamy pâtés. Glorious wedges of Brie. Big juicy steaks.

Those are not low-budget items.

And what about all those fancy cocktail parties fast-laners like to hold and attend? You can pack over a thousand calories into a single raid on an hors-d'oeuvres tray. And cocktails themselves are *very* fattening.

It's one of life's bitterest ironies: At a time when your wallet can most afford the foods you've learned to love, your body can least afford to absorb them without leaving nasty bumps and bulges.

What about the cheap treats? We're talking fast foods. Hamburgers and fries, double malteds, carryout chicken wings—they all spell trouble.

We subject ourselves to excess stress—and stress leads to overeating.

Our culture has trained us to eat our troubles away. Having a hard afternoon? Gobble a candy bar! Feeling blue? Try a cheesecake pick-me-up! Need a treat? Go out for a big dinner!

Try this instead: The next time you're feeling wired, go for what Dr. Herbert Benson labels the "relaxation response." Find yourself a comfortable sitting position. Close your eyes. Relax every muscle in your body, starting with your toes and working up to your head—or the other way around. Then empty your mind of everything except a clear, bright focus on your breathing.

Inhale slowly and deeply. Exhale slowly: Each time you do, think (or say softly) the word "one."

When distracting thoughts come knocking at your consciousness, let them in—and let them out again. Don't pay them any attention. With practice, you'll find out what a clear head means.

Keep this up for from fifteen to twenty minutes or until you feel terrific.

Yes, this *is* a form of meditation, but don't let it scare you. All I know is this: It's a whole lot healthier than a shot of sugar, and I've never heard of anyone crashing afterward.

THE FAST LANE DIET

Our days are so full that there's no room for regular exercise.

There's that old problem, time, again. We simply don't have enough of it to set aside an hour for a brisk walk or a trip to the health club or a racquetball game or an aerobics workout at the Y.

For now, suffice it to say that no diet can do it all. If you sit in a chair for five straight weeks and consume 200 calories a day, at the end of that time you'll have lost weight—but you'll look as if you've been sitting in a chair for five straight weeks.

Here's some good news: The Fast Lane Diet is going to give you time you didn't know you had. How? By making it completely unnecessary for you to search out restaurants that feature diet lunches or to weigh foods when preparing meals at home or to take hours fixing fancy "diet foods."

The Fast Lane Diet is the *only* diet I know of that fits in with the fast lane lifestyle. It's simple, portable, delicious, nutritionally sound—and you make the drink in a *hurry*, gaining *extra* time to get out and tone those rapidly emerging muscles and lean limbs.

It's likely that you've got a lot of years ahead of you. And though you're not going to get any younger, chronologically speaking, you can start *feeling* younger today by shedding those extra pounds.

That's what the Fast Lane Diet is for. It worked for me; it can work for you, too.

4

THE FAST LANE DIET DRINK: The Basic Recipe Plus Thirty-one Variations

The Basic Recipe

Here are some things you should know about the Fast Lane Diet Drink.

It costs only 20 cents per serving, up to $3 less than any commercially prepared formulas, many of which contain chemicals.

It can be made ahead and frozen for later use.

It is totally sound nutritionally.

It satisfies the appetite for from three to four hours.

It is made at home with all-natural ingredients. It's even great for children.

The Fast Lane Diet Drink is the key to the fast lane way of shedding pounds and keeping trim.

The Fast Lane Diet Drink will not interrupt your lifestyle! Used in conjunction with one of the six Fast Lane Diets offered in this book, this drink is a totally nutritious, totally portable, totally delicious beverage that will fit right in with your fast lane way of life.

■ *The Basic Recipe for the Fast Lane Diet Drink*

   3 cups dry skim milk powder

   4 cups water

   4 teaspoons corn oil

   2 teaspoons vanilla extract

   2 packets artificial sweetener (optional)

   Combine ingredients in a 1-quart pitcher and stir thoroughly.

The basic Diet Drink recipe makes four servings of the Fast Lane Diet Drink. If you want to make only two servings, just divide the recipe in half. Each serving of the Fast Lane Diet Drink contains 220 calories.

When it's time for your Diet Drink, all you do is pour one cup of the Diet Drink into a blender, food processor, or shaker. Add six crushed ice cubes and blend for a really frothy drink. It isn't necessary to "shake up" the Diet Drink, but it does make the drink taste more like a milk shake, and most people prefer it that way.

Plus Thirty-one Variations

The basic Fast Lane Diet Drink is absolutely delicious as is but can be varied by adding all kinds of fruits and other flavorings.

Here are thirty-one delicious variations and the calorie count of each. For each drink, just whirl in a blender and eat with a spoon. If your basic recipe contains artificial sweetener, you needn't use it in those of the following recipes that include it. Don't put it in twice!

■ **Banana Drink**

1 cup Diet Drink

½ banana

½ teaspoon cinnamon

6 ice cubes, crushed

270 calories

■ **Blueberry Drink**

1 cup Diet Drink

½ cup blueberries

1 teaspoon cinnamon

6 crushed ice cubes

265 calories

■ **Chocolate Shake**

1 cup Diet Drink (unsweetened)

1 package sugar-free cocoa mix

6 crushed ice cubes

270 calories

■ **Grape Drink**

1 cup Diet Drink

½ cup halved green seedless grapes

½ teaspoon coconut extract

6 crushed ice cubes

270 calories

■ **Piña Colada Drink**

1 cup Diet Drink

½ teaspoon coconut extract

½ banana

6 crushed ice cubes

270 calories

■ *Peach Mocha*

1 cup Diet Drink (unsweetened)

½ large fresh peach, sliced, or 6 slices frozen or canned
   unsweetened peaches

½ teaspoon cinnamon

1 tablespoon instant coffee

6 crushed ice cubes

½ package sugar-free cocoa mix

265 calories

■ *Jogger's Drink*

¾ cup Diet Drink (unsweetened)

1 egg

½ package sugar-free cocoa mix

250 calories

■ *Banana Strawberry Drink*

1 cup Diet Drink

½ banana

3 fresh or frozen strawberries

6 crushed ice cubes

270 calories

■ *Soda Drink*

1 cup Diet Drink (unsweetened)

½ cup any flavor diet soda

6 crushed ice cubes

220 calories

■ *Apple Coconut Drink*

1 cup Diet Drink

½ apple, sliced

½ teaspoon coconut extract

1 teaspoon lemon juice

6 crushed ice cubes

260 calories

■ **Cola Drink**

1 cup Diet Drink

½ fresh peach or 6 frozen or canned
  unsweetened peach slices

½ cup diet cola

6 crushed ice cubes

260 calories

■ **Melon Drink**

1 cup Diet Drink

1 cup cantaloupe or honeydew chunks

1½ teaspoons lemon juice

6 crushed ice cubes

268 calories

■ **The Peach Lifter**

1 cup Diet Drink

½ cored and sliced apple

½ large fresh peach or 6 frozen or canned
  unsweetened peach slices

1 squirt of fresh lime juice

6 crushed ice cubes

270 calories

■ **Hawaiian Drink**

1 cup Diet Drink

½ teaspoon coconut extract

¼ cup crushed pineapple (unsweetened)

■ *Hawaiian Drink* (continued)

1 tablespoon frozen orange juice concentrate

3 fresh or frozen strawberries

6 crushed ice cubes

285 calories

■ *Eye Opener*

1 cup Diet Drink

1 tablespoon orange juice concentrate

¼ cup crushed pineapple (unsweetened)

½ sliced fresh peach or 6 frozen or canned
unsweetened peach slices

6 crushed ice cubes

275 calories

■ *Northerner's Delight*

1 cup Diet Drink

½ teaspoon maple extract

½ cored and sliced fresh apple

6 crushed ice cubes

260 calories

■ *Tutti-Frutti*

1 cup Diet Drink

½ fresh peach or 6 slices frozen or canned
unsweetened peaches

¼ cup fresh or frozen blueberries

½ teaspoon coconut extract

6 crushed ice cubes

253 calories

■ *Pentathlon Special*

1 cup Diet Drink

½ fresh peach or 6 frozen or canned
   unsweetened peach slices

½ cored and sliced apple

1 tablespoon frozen orange juice concentrate

6 crushed ice cubes

290 calories

■ *Key Lime Frost*

1 cup Diet Drink (unsweetened)

1 teaspoon fresh lemon juice

1 teaspoon fresh lime juice

1 packet artificial sweetener

6 crushed ice cubes

230 calories

■ *Pineapple Upside-Down Drink*

1 cup Diet Drink (unsweetened)

4 fresh or canned unsweetened pineapple chunks

¼ teaspoon cinnamon

½ banana

1 packet artificial sweetener

6 crushed ice cubes

290 calories

■ *Peppermint Delight*

1 cup Diet Drink

¼ teaspoon peppermint extract

6 crushed ice cubes

245 calories

■ **Banana Rum Punch**

   1 cup Diet Drink (unsweetened)

   ¼ teaspoon rum-flavored extract

   ½ banana

   1 packet artificial sweetener

   6 crushed ice cubes

   270 calories

■ **Tart Raspberry Drink**

   1 cup Diet Drink (unsweetened)

   ½ cup fresh or frozen unsweetened raspberries

   1 squirt fresh lemon juice

   1 packet artificial sweetener

   6 crushed ice cubes

   261 calories

■ **Coffee Lover's Drink**

   1 cup Diet Drink

   1 teaspoon instant coffee

   ½ banana

   6 crushed ice cubes

   270 calories

■ **Banana Chocolate Drink**

   1 cup Diet Drink (unsweetened)

   ½ package sugar-free cocoa mix

   ½ banana

   1 packet artificial sweetener

   6 crushed ice cubes

   295 calories

■ *Brandied Peaches*

1 cup Diet Drink

½ fresh peach, peeled and sliced or 6 frozen or canned unsweetened peach slices

¼ teaspoon brandy extract

6 crushed ice cubes

260 calories

■ *Watermelon Drink*

1 cup Diet Drink

1 cup chunked watermelon

1 teaspoon cinnamon

6 crushed ice cubes

262 calories

■ *Almond Shake*

1 cup Diet Drink

½ teaspoon almond extract

½ banana

6 crushed ice cubes

270 calories

■ *Carob Drink*

1 cup Diet Drink

1 teaspoon cinnamon

1 tablespoon carob powder

6 crushed ice cubes

275 calories

■ **Root Beer Float**

1 cup Diet Drink

½ cup diet root beer

6 crushed ice cubes

220 calories

■ **Café au Lait**

½ cup hot Diet Drink (yes, you can heat it, too)

½ cup hot espresso or very strong coffee

½ teaspoon almond extract

160 calories

Fresh or Frozen?

If fresh fruits are available, *use them*! If they aren't, it's better to substitute frozen than canned fruits. Frozen fruits tend to be more flavorful and are less likely to be laden with sweetened syrup. If you must use canned fruit, be certain you use fruit that's packed in its own juices. The last thing you want to do is add calories to the Diet Drink.

I usually *partially* freeze fresh fruit before adding it to the basic Fast Lane Diet Drink recipe. I find that fruit that's partially frozen cuts up better and makes for a thicker, richer drink. To freeze bananas, peel them first; then freeze them in plastic bags. I usually have a supply on hand since so many of the Diet Drinks rely on them.

It's a good idea to prepare several batches of the basic Diet Drink recipe and then freeze one-serving portions for later use. When you are ready to use one, just add whatever fruit you've got a yen for.

Freeze individual servings of the basic Diet Drink to take with you on vacations or when you're on the run—and that's most of the time, isn't it?

You are always free to improvise! Just build on the basic Diet

Drink recipe. Stick to fresh, natural, low-calorie ingredients, and you can't go wrong.

Don't Take That Oil from the Fast Lane Drink

The oil in the Fast Lane Diet Drink is a very important ingredient. Here's why:

Oil contains lecithin, which is essential to your body.

Oil contains Vitamin E.

Having oil in the diet gives a feeling of fullness. You aren't likely to get hungry as quickly. Eating 100 calories of oil can prevent you from eating 500 calories of another food because it is satisfying.

Lack of fat in the diet causes you to become very hungry. You know what happens then—you develop cravings for rich, fattening food.

Lack of fat causes your blood sugar to plunge, making you feel sick.

For Those Cruising in the Low-Calcium Lane

Here's an added benefit for Fast Lane Diet Drink users: The Diet Drink contains a large amount of calcium. When used in conjunction with one of the six Fast Lane Diet programs, this drink provides the user with extra calcium protection. This is especially important for the following fast-laners:

- Pregnant women. No doubt you have been advised by your doctor that you need extra calcium for yourself and your unborn baby.

- Women in their late thirties to early forties. Recent studies suggest that women who take extra calcium in the years before menopause are less likely to develop osteoporosis, a gradual weakening of the bones that is a direct result of calcium deficiency.

- Nursing mothers. The extra supply of calcium in the Fast Lane Diet Drink is a great boost for nursing mothers who don't like to drink plain milk.

- Kids. Even if they don't like milk, they may love the taste of the Fast Lane Diet Drink because it tastes so much like a milk shake.

How to Get High Fiber in the Fast Lane Diet

We're all becoming increasingly fiber-conscious, especially since recent studies have linked a low-fiber diet with developing certain forms of cancer.

Fiber is the indigestible part of plant food. It has no nutritional value, cannot be absorbed by the body, and does not supply calories.

Why is it useful? It adds bulk to your diet because of its water-absorbing ability. It takes food through your body quickly and efficiently. It is absolutely necessary for proper bowel functioning. It is found in fruits and vegetables, in seeds and nuts, and in whole grain flours, cereals, and breads made from whole grain ingredients.

The Fast Lane Diet is high in fiber when natural fruit is added to the Diet Drink. It is for this reason that I absolutely recommend that all fast-laners have *at least one fruity version of the Diet Drink per day.*

I also recommend that fast-laners supplement *each of the diet plans* with several glasses of water daily. If you have trouble remembering to drink water, keep a handsome crystal decanter on the kitchen counter or on your office desk at all times. It's an attractive reminder.

Now read on and see how the Fast Lane Diet Drink fits into six different diet plans.

5

WHICH FAST LANE DIET IS RIGHT FOR YOU? A Twenty-Question Quiz

One of the things you, as a fast-laner, are really going to love about this diet is that it gives you a choice. There isn't just one type of fast lane lifestyle—and, likewise, there isn't just one Fast Lane Diet. There are six—and you can use the one that best suits your current needs. If your needs change, just switch to a different Fast Lane Diet. No doubt, as a member of the fast lane, you've learned how to turn on a dime.

To find the Fast Lane Diet that's right for you *right now*, take the following twenty-question quiz. It shouldn't take more than a half hour of your valuable time, but it's well worth it because it will lead you right to your diet plan.

1. How do you feel about your present weight?
    A. I'm at least 5 pounds overweight, and I'm willing to take the weight off at a moderate pace.
    B. I have at least 5 pounds to lose, but I'm never happy following a diet.

C. I have a small amount of weight to lose, and I'd like to see it drop off quickly.

D. My extra weight's been creeping up on me for a long time, so I guess although I know I have to lose it, I want to do it slowly—I need a diet that will fit into my schedule.

E. I'm always on one diet or another. I guess I'm as addicted to diets as I am to food.

F. I've already lost weight, and I'm where I want to be. I'd like to maintain my present weight without making changes in my lifestyle.

2. The following statement describes my lifestyle.

A. I'm a fast-laner, all right, but I do usually have at least one meal a day at a table—lunch or dinner.

B. I'm the fastest fast-laner I know. I'm so busy that I rarely take time to prepare a meal for myself.

C. It varies. I can alter my schedule to suit my fast lane needs.

D. I have a nonstop day but often have a business lunch or dinner.

E. I'm always on the go and rarely have time for a real sit-down meal.

F. I'm a fast-laner, all right, but I've learned how to moderate my eating habits to make the most of my life.

3. How do you feel about eating alone?

A. I can eat two meals a day alone, but I like company for at least one meal a day, usually dinner.

B. I don't like eating alone, but I'm usually on the run, and I'm not big on cooking for myself, so I often do eat alone.

C. It's OK with me. If I need to do something in order to look and feel better, then I just do it—even if it means doing it alone.

D. I don't really get much chance to eat alone. At lunch I'm always conducting business, and at dinner I'm either socially obligated or grabbing time to be with the family.

E. I don't think of it as eating alone. I think of it more as eating anonymously since so much of it is done while I'm standing up, walking from place to place, or telephoning.

F. I prefer not to eat alone, but I've been on a lot of diets and have learned to do whatever is necessary to keep my weight down.

4. How do you feel about lunch?

A. I'm always hungry at lunchtime, but I get even hungrier as the day wears on. I'm usually ravenous by dinner.

B. Lunch is not an event for me, but I'll eat plenty of whatever it is I can get.

C. When I eat lunch out, I really enjoy eating a special meal in a good restaurant; otherwise, I'm content with whatever's available.

D. I have big lunches because I usually do business over lunch. It's often my biggest meal of the day.

E. It's no more important than any other meal since I have a tendency to eat and "pick" all day long.

F. I try to take time to eat a balanced lunch. I know it's an important meal and have learned to eat nutritionally even if I eat in a hurry.

5. What has your weight history been?

A. I've always watched my weight for as long as I can remember. Lately I'm weighing in higher than I used to and find myself counting calories when I'm in a restaurant.

B. I'm usually watching my weight because I have a tendency to eat a lot of junk foods that are high in calories. I don't have the best eating habits.

C. I'm usually pretty close to my desired weight, but every so often the extra pounds creep on—and then I need to diet to take them off again.

D. I've been overweight since I embarked on my Fast Lane lifestyle, which requires that I eat while I work. The extra business cocktail before lunch doesn't help either.

E. Up and down. I'm like a yo-yo, gaining and losing, binging and dieting.

F. I've recently found a way to get my weight down where I want it to be. Now I'm looking for a way to keep it there—permanently.

6. How do you feel about exercise?

A. I follow an exercise program that works well with my fast lane lifestyle. It isn't always easy to make time for it, but I know it's important.

B. I'm so busy that I rarely have time for exercise.

C. I exercise in spurts. I guess you could say I go through periods when I'm serious about my exercise program and periods when I don't exercise at all.

D. My exercise often involves business—like taking a client to dine at the club or to play golf.

E. The best exercise I get is nonstop movement. I walk a lot—unless, of course, I happen to be running.

F. I've found an exercise program that works for my lifestyle. I exercise pretty religiously; if I didn't, I'd probably gain weight.

7. When do you get hungriest?

A. Throughout the day because I need food just to keep me going through my fast lane paces. I find my hunger increases proportionately with my fast lane pace.

B. As the day goes on, especially toward the evening. I sometimes eat without being especially hungry.

C. I go on binges, and then I can go for two or three days without feeling hungry at all.

D. At lunchtime—mostly because I'm conditioned to having my main meal of the day then.

E. All day long. I tend to nibble throughout the day.

F. Even more, it seems, when I'm dieting and really watching my weight.

8. How do you feel about diets?

A. They are a necessary evil. I don't love following them, of course, but I'm willing to do so.

B. Most of them require too much weighing and measuring and shopping. I just don't have the time.

C. Most of them take too long to see results.

D. Many of them just aren't compatible with my hectic lifestyle. I have a hard time following them in restaurants.

E. They require too much time investment in sit-down meals. I'm often eating on the run.

F. They don't help you sustain weight loss. They get you there—but they aren't a program you can follow for a long period of time.

9. What is your biggest food problem?

A. I'm finding it increasingly difficult to keep weight off while following my busy-as-ever, fast lane lifestyle.

B. I don't have enough time to prepare nutritionally sound menus for myself or my family.

C. I love to binge and then regret it later on.

D. I have to eat in restaurants all the time. It's an important part of the way I do business.

E. I nibble all day long, rarely taking the time to eat meals.

F. I don't want to give up the foods I like to eat, but I do want to stay healthy and slim.

10. If you were handed a dinner menu, you would probably select the following:

   A. roast beef, au gratin potatoes, apple pie.

   B. cheeseburger, french fries, and a milk shake.

   C. duck with orange sauce, wild rice, chocolate mousse.

   D. steak, Caesar salad, and cheesecake.

   E. assorted appetizers, soup, sherbet.

   F. halibut, broccoli with cheese sauce, strawberries with whipped cream.

11. Do you eat out a lot?

   A. Only when necessary. With my fast lane lifestyle, I can't avoid eating out occasionally, but I do try to eat at least one main meal (breakfast or lunch) at home each day.

   B. I seem to do it a great deal. Not in fancy restaurants—more in the fast-food variety.

   C. In good restaurants. I try to do it at least twice a week, but it isn't necessarily a part of my daily lifestyle.

   D. I eat lunch out at least three times a week—my profession demands that I do business at lunch.

   E. I eat out, in, everywhere, and anywhere that I find myself—at all times of the day.

   F. Yes. But I'd rather prepare my own meals and know what's going into them.

12. How often are you in the kitchen?

   A. A lot. Especially near the refrigerator.

   B. Rarely. I'm not really into cooking—maybe I would be if I had more time.

   C. Every so often. I'll go through periods when I'm doing a lot of cooking and periods where I'm just making do with whatever's in the refrigerator.

   D. Hardly at all. My biggest meal of the day is lunch in a restaurant, and I don't eat much in the evenings.

E. A lot. I snack all the time, so when I'm home, the kitchen seems to be where I spend most of my time.

F. As often as I need to be to maintain my weight at the proper level.

13. How important is your appearance to you?

A. Very important, especially now, because I'm beginning to realize that I will not be able to keep myself attractive unless I work at it a bit—I'm not getting any younger.

B. Quite important, but I don't have time to fuss much over the way I look.

C. Very important, and I'll do just about anything to see that I remain attractive.

D. I think a lot about my image—the way I present myself in my career. It's important to look good in the fast lane.

E. Important, but I know I'd look and feel much better if I ate foods that were more nutritious.

F. It always has been important, and now that I look and feel really good, I'm concerned about staying fit.

14. How many meals do you like to eat?

A. I like to have three square ones a day—even though I'm incredibly busy.

B. I like to have three meals a day, but they're often rushed and gobbled down.

C. I don't have to be conventional in the three-meals-a-day sense; I'm aware of nutrition, so I feel OK as long as I'm getting enough of the so-called right foods.

D. I usually do have breakfast and lunch. Dinner I could really take or leave because I'm not as hungry then; sometimes I eat it without wanting to.

E. I think I used to eat real meals—way back when. Now that I'm really in the fast lane, I just don't have time.

F. I used to be more hurried about my meals. Now I

usually take the time out of my busy schedule to eat at least two square meals a day.

15. How is your health?

A. I feel a whole lot better when I'm thinner than I am right now.

B. It worries me. I know my whirlwind lifestyle isn't adding years to my life.

C. Pretty good—I try to keep in shape and pay attention to my body's signals.

D. It could be better. I feel especially sluggish after a big business lunch and don't work as well some afternoons as I should. I fall asleep earlier than I used to and need coffee to get me going in the morning.

E. OK. I really don't have much time to think about it, though.

F. Probably a lot better these days because I've been paying attention to my diet more than I used to. I'd like to stay healthy without having to live in health food stores—I don't have time to devote myself to a radical change in lifestyle.

16. How would you describe your family?

A. Demanding of my time. Not that I don't love and care about them—I want to give them as much of myself as I possibly can.

B. Understanding. Whatever everyone eats is OK with them. We're a modern family, I guess, and we're *all* in the fast lane.

C. Weight- and health-conscious even though we're all fast-laners.

D. Wonderful, but it seems as if I hardly see them these days.

E. Incredibly busy. We're all on a treadmill, leaving notes on the refrigerator and dashing out the door.

F. A lot happier when I'm happier. They like to see me taking care of myself.

17. How do you feel about food?

    A. It's a shame I can't eat as much of it as I want without worrying about my weight.

    B. It's something you need to keep you going—it's definitely *not* the most important thing in my life.

    C. It's wonderful when you have the time really to enjoy it; otherwise, it's just something you need to keep you active and healthy.

    D. I've learned to enjoy a wide variety of foods in a wide variety of restaurants. I like ethnic foods and enjoy a gourmet meal.

    E. I want to eat all day long and seem to crave certain types of foods—salty, sweet, and greasy. My food needs can be pretty specific and pretty obsessive.

    F. I've learned to control my interest in food and am realistic about my food needs.

18. Do you want to change your eating pattern?

    A. No. I need a diet that fits in with my and my family's lifestyle.

    B. I guess . . . I really don't think I *have* any pattern.

    C. Sure, but I feel more comfortable if I'm not asked to follow an eating "program" day in and day out.

    D. Impossible. I have to eat big business lunches!

    E. What eating pattern? I don't think I've had one for a long time now.

    F. Sure, if it's going to keep my weight down. Still, I'd like to alter my lifestyle as little as possible.

19. Why did you buy this book?

    A. I've been eating the same as always—but for the last few years I've been fighting the battle of the bulge. I have to take off this extra weight, but I don't want to make changes in my lifestyle—and other diets don't seem to fit in with my fast pace.

    B. I'm sick and tired of diets that require me to weigh,

measure, and eat three big meals a day at the table—
I simply don't have the time!

C. I have some extra weight I want to take off quickly.

D. I consider myself a real fast-laner and can't believe
there's a diet that will actually fill my needs.

E. I'm desperate. I've tried diet after diet, but I always
gain back the weight I've lost. I'm definitely in the
fast lane and don't have time for other diet programs.

F. I weigh what I want to weigh—so I really need a
lifelong diet that fits in with my lifestyle—I don't want
to be a chronic dieter.

20. How would you describe your ideal diet?

A. A diet that isn't too specific so that I can eat the main
meal whenever I have the time to prepare it.

B. One that allows me to eat foods that are readily available—and not foods that have to be prepared by me.

C. One that I can go on for a couple of days—then go
back to my regular eating pattern.

D. One that allows me the freedom of eating out in restaurants—I wish more of them would offer diet menus.

E. One that allows me to eat snack foods and nibble food
throughout the day.

F. A diet I can live with *daily* without really feeling as if
I am on a diet.

Now tally your responses. If you have mostly A's, turn to
the answer key and read the description of type A; mostly B's,
read type B; and so on. The type of fast-laner you are will
determine which diet plan you should follow.

Type A

If you've chosen mostly A's, you're ready for the regular Fast
Lane Diet program. This is the original Fast Lane Diet—the

one that gave birth to all the others. It's not an irresponsible crash diet, but you can expect to lose between 3 and 8 pounds the first week and somewhat less the second, depending on how much weight you have to lose. In the process, you should gain an awareness of what it means to be a fast-laner and realize that moderating your fast lane lifestyle can afford you all kinds of benefits.

The original Fast Lane Diet is a program for fast-laners who are aware they need to pay more attention to basic nutrition, but haven't the foggiest notion of how to go about doing so while still remaining a member in good standing of the fast lane.

Type A's are on a whirlwind course. Up until now, that's been OK for you. But now there's a big signpost in the road that says, *"Hold everything."* Sure, you're going great guns, and you're more successful than you've ever been before. Sure, you're getting patted on the back by just about everyone, and the rewards for being a go-getter are tangible. But what are you losing while you're gaining all this self-esteem? What is success in the fast lane costing you?

You probably picked up this book because you're willing to accept the fact that it may be time for a change. What you are about to learn is that the change needn't be radical. If you use the Fast Lane Diet Drink as a dietary supplement in combination with a basic good-sense eating program, you're bound to see results.

As I've said, weight loss will not be dramatic, but it will be relatively painless, and it will not, I repeat *not*, interfere with your fast lane lifestyle.

So, all you type A's, get with it. What you need to realize is that you're overweight *because* you're a member in good standing of the fast lane, and what you're gaining in status and bank balance you're losing in terms of your overall health. You also need to understand that you don't have to alter your lifestyle dramatically in order to shed pounds. It's as easy to be a healthy fast-laner as it is to be a tired, overweight fast-laner.

Now turn your attention to Chapter 7 and the original Fast Lane Diet.

* * *

Type B

Congratulations! You're in the passing lane, and that means you're moving faster than anyone else on the road. Maybe you have more than one job, or you're in night school, or you spend long hours—even weekends—at the office because you have so much to accomplish and the days aren't getting any longer. Maybe you're angling for a better, higher-paying position, or maybe you're already there and you intend to stay there. Or maybe you have four kids under the age of six!

Being in the passing lane is an exhausting experience, and if you're there for any amount of time, you deserve the Survival Medal of Honor. I know. I was there.

But I'm not here to tell you to give up that exciting pace. Most passing-laners are people who need to rely on fast-food restaurants and barely have time to grab a hot dog or prepare a frozen dinner. Well, on the Passing Lane Diet, that's exactly what type B's do.

In Chapter 8, discover the Passing Lane Diet. See how it's possible to thrive on the insanity of your lifestyle and still lose weight.

Type C

If you're a type C, you probably haven't been surprised by what's been said so far in this book. For some time now you've known all about the sacrifices you're making in order to be in the fast lane. But you're a savvy fast-laner. You're willing to compensate for your fast lane existence—and you're probably already engaging in some form of physical activity on a regular basis. You know something about diet and nutrition and try to stick to salads and steer clear of fatty foods. Perhaps you even venture into a health store when you have the time. Maybe you're a runner. Or you work out. You have tried, in other words, to find a way to take care of yourself while you exult in being in the fast lane.

But don't pat yourself on the back—at least not yet. After all, you bought this book, didn't you? That means that as much as you think you know, you're still searching for a diet program that fits in with your lifestyle. You probably don't need the original Fast Lane Diet (a two-week program), but you do have some weight to lose and you want dramatic results and a program that's easy to follow.

I think you'll appreciate the Fast Lane Fast. If you've put on some extra pounds and you want to lose them in a hurry, the Fast Lane Fast is the simplest of diets—and the shortest. If you follow it for just three days, you can expect to lose as much as 8 pounds!

The Fast Lane Fast is, like most fasts, something of a cleansing. It's a great diet to go on after a vacation, after the holidays, after the weekend, after a round of entertaining. Type C's are perhaps the most flexible of fast-laners, willing to starve themselves when necessary so they can indulge themselves during other times. But guess what? You don't have to starve. You can still make the sacrifice, take off the extra pounds quickly, and continue to live your fast lane life to the fullest.

I use the Fast Lane Fast whenever I feel just a bit heavier than I want to be. I feel that it not only gives my body a rest but it also lifts my spirits! Some people think I'm doing penance for having indulged. I prefer to think of the Fast Lane Fast as a great gift I am giving myself—something like a day at a health spa or a weekend in the country. Every so often even the most ardent fast-laner needs a breather.

To learn more about the Fast Lane Fast, turn to Chapter 9.

Type D

If you've answered mostly D's, you're in the fast lane, and you're proud of it. It's taken you quite a while to accomplish what you have, and you wouldn't give up your elevated fast lane lifestyle for anything. The problem is that to remain at the top you have to eat out a great deal—business lunches and dinners—and that means choosing among menus containing many high-calorie dishes.

It's certainly difficult to stay on a diet while your lunch date is drowning in fettuccine Alfredo and martinis. But there are fast lane fields that require business lunches or dinners as part of the daily game—for example, advertising, law, publishing, television, film. If you get to choose the restaurant, you can pick Chinese over Italian or French for lower-calorie choices. But you don't want your lunch partner to feel guilty, do you? So you go right ahead and order spare ribs with black bean sauce even though the moo goo gai pan would have done nicely. You can find fattening foods in *any* restaurant, and when they're right there on that mouth-watering menu, they're awfully hard to resist.

If you're an executive business-luncher, chances are you've been at the mercy of the gourmet menu for years. But the Fast Lane Business Lunch Diet offers all type D's a lifeline.

Turn to Chapter 10 to see how it's possible to do lunch and still stay fast lane trim.

Type E

If you've chosen mostly E's, the On-the-Road Diet is just right for you. This one is for two types of fast-laners: the snackers—who just plain love to nibble all day long—and the grazers—those who are, for one reason or another, just too busy to sit down to meals.

The snackers may be housewives or lawyers or doctors or college professors; if you're one, you know you don't always eat the right foods. The snackers often get food cravings and may want to eat one type of food for days—chocolate, sunflower seeds, popcorn. Snackers eat throughout the day, at no special time. They often find themselves eating their small meals in odd places—over a sink, over a desk, on a train platform, in a car.

The grazers are snackers who just don't find the time to sit down to meals. Grazers are often victims of their own busy schedules. It's not that they adore snack foods; it's just that snack foods seem to them the only foods that are portable. Snack foods can be purchased while waiting for a bus and can be eaten while walking to or from a meeting. Grazers especially like food that is filling, energy-producing, and quick. I see grazers in parks, on street corners, and in the lobbies of major office buildings. They're a multiplying breed.

If you're a snacker or a grazer, you probably think there isn't a diet on earth that will allow you the freedom, portability, or flexibility you need. Think again. The On-the-Road Diet offers all that and more.

Turn to Chapter 11 for the snacking-good truth.

Type F

I'm not crazy about the word "maintenance," because the last thing I, as a fast-laner, want is something that requires even more of my time and energy. Maintenance sounds like work, and the Staying-on-Course Diet is as easy to follow as its five counterparts.

A word fast-laners *do* feel comfortable with is "transition" because all fast-laners are in a constant state of growth and transition. That's what being in the fast lane is all about.

The Staying-on-Course Diet is a transitional diet—a two-week program that allows you to ease gradually into a normal, healthy eating pattern. If you've selected mostly F's, the chances are that you've lost weight and you'd like to keep it off. You've learned something about nutrition, but you're afraid that if you start eating again the way you used to, you're likely to gain back all the weight you lost. But you don't want to stay on a diet the rest of your life either!

On the Staying-on-Course Diet, you'll gradually increase your food intake via a two-week program of sensible eating supplemented by the Fast Lane Diet Drink. After two weeks of "transition," you will—we hope—have learned a great deal about proper nutrition, and you will be using your new knowledge to its best advantage. You will have learned, for example, that being busy doesn't mean you have to eat poorly or eat nothing but fattening fast foods. You will have learned that even on your crazy schedule it is possible to follow a program of healthy eating—and keep your weight down right where you want it to be.

Turn to Chapter 12 and learn how to stay on course.

6

PROFILES OF FAST-LANERS:
Is One of Them You?

Dieting can be a lonely business. If you've taken the quiz, found your diet, and are about to embark on the Fast Lane Diet without a friend, it may help you to identify with some fast-laners who've been on the road before you.

Here are six profiles of fast-laners—one for each Fast Lane Diet. Each profile contains a before and after: before and after the Fast Lane Diet. If reading the profile of your fast lane type makes you feel right at home, you'll know you're on the right track and may even feel more optimistic about the rewards of the diet you've chosen.

Type A Fast-Laner

NAME: Charlie
AGE: Middle fifties
OCCUPATION: Corporation president

No one ever doubted that Charlie would rise to the top of his field. He was senior class president, editor of the school news-paper, in the top ten of his college graduating class—you name it. His high school friends remember him as the one they voted "most likely to succeed." They were right. By the age of 30, Charlie had already been named vice president of a Fortune 500 company. At 38 he was named president and is next in line to be chairman of the board.

Somewhere along the way, Charlie found the time to get married, have four children, take up golf, and get into a satisfying but sporadic jogging program. In a typical day Charlie would be up at 5:30, off for a morning jog, and on to the office by 8:00.

A big part of Charlie's week was the board meeting. Usually these meetings coincided with eating since they often lasted through the lunch period. Lunch was usually brought in, and since it took too long for each person to order separately, one person ordered for everyone. There were deli sandwiches, soda, coffee or milk, and cookies or cake for dessert.

Then it was home by 6:00, where Charlie tried to be on time for the family meal. He really treasured the time he spent at home with his wife, Catherine, and his four daughters, who ranged in age from 6 to 15. Catherine was an excellent cook and prepared lovely family meals.

One day Charlie checked his weight after his morning jog around the park. While he had noticed that his clothes were not as comfortable as they had been, he was surprised to see that he had gained nearly 20 pounds in a little over a year.

Charlie was shocked. He'd thought his jogging and his occasional golf game would keep his weight from really getting away from him. Obviously, he'd been wrong.

In the days that followed, Charlie noticed that he also felt somewhat sluggish and that he was becoming tired during meetings and felt like going home early night after night. When he mentioned his concern to Catherine, she said that she had noticed that he had put on some weight but hadn't said anything for fear of hurting his feelings.

Now that Charlie was asking for help, she was ready to give it. She knew about the Fast Lane Diet Drink, so she decided to make up a batch. She and Charlie loved the flavor, so they both went on the original Fast Lane Diet program.

Charlie was able to get through those fattening board meeting lunches because he brought his Fast Lane Diet Drink of the day with him and found it was every bit as satisfying as the deli sandwiches and soda. In the evenings, he and Catherine had a Fast Lane Diet dinner together; the girls enjoyed it, too.

After the two-week program, Charlie and Catherine went on a program of moderate eating, supplemented by the Fast Lane Diet Drink, which had become a daily ritual. Even their daughters loved the drink, and Catherine made it up in big batches that she froze for later use.

Charlie is confident that he'll be able to maintain his weight because he now weighs himself regularly. If he gains a pound or two, he resorts to the Fast Lane Diet to set him back on course. He feels he has found a diet plan that fits in perfectly with the way he lives and the way he works.

Type B Fast-Laner

NAME: Chris
AGE: 32
OCCUPATION: Homemaker and mother of three

After each of her children was born, Chris gained 10 pounds. With the birth of Melissa, her third child, Chris was clearly 30 pounds overweight, not to mention overwrought, exhausted, and without a clue as to how to lose the weight she'd gained. Her body shape had changed along with the weight gain. But frantic day-to-day life with a 4-year-old, a 3-year-old, and a 1½-year-old didn't give Chris much of a chance even to think about dieting.

With three kids, Chris noticed, she was preparing four to five meals a day (not counting an evening meal that she and her husband, Steve, tried to have at least five nights a week) and was cleaning up after the kids' meals by eating what they left behind. What mother hasn't done that? In addition, she was eating some of all of the meals she was preparing and then having an evening meal with Steve!

One day Steve came home with two tickets to London for their fifth wedding anniversary. He'd planned to surprise her, but he had thought better about it since there was so much preparation involved in making the trip. So he scheduled their trip for the first week of June, giving Chris two months to get ready.

Chris became frantic. Apart from all the packing and child-care plans, she didn't fit into any of her nonmaternity clothes. Steve had given her $1,000 to shop for some new clothes to take to Europe.

Chris was determined not to buy any new clothes in America *or* Europe in fat sizes. But what could she do? She didn't have much time what with getting Steve and herself ready for the trip and taking care of the day-to-day business of bringing up the kids. She was busier than ever now and had no time to engage in an intricate, time-absorbing diet plan or to embark on a new exercise program.

Then one day her son's nursery school teacher told her about the Fast Lane Diet. Chris loved the Fast Lane Diet Drink from the moment she tasted it and began using it in conjunction with the Passing Lane Diet. At first she felt guilty preparing convenience foods for Steve, but he assured her that he didn't mind at all; in fact, it took some of the pressure off him to be home in time for a dinner he knew she'd so painstakingly prepared.

Chris lost nearly 15 pounds on the Passing Lane Diet in just three weeks and still relies on the Fast Lane Diet Drink to get her through the day. She's certain it will remain a part of her eating pattern for the rest of her life.

Type C Fast-Laner

NAME: Terri
AGE: 26
OCCUPATION: Flight attendant

As flight attendant for a major international airline, Terri always had to look her best on the job. She had always been very weight-conscious. Although she'd always looked like a natural beauty, she had actually worked hard at maintaining her striking good looks.

Her boyfriend, a pilot named Greg, was also a real fast-laner, and so were the three other flight attendants Terri lived with. They never kept a lot of food in the refrigerator because no one knew who would be home to eat it or when. They tended to eat mostly on the run, and it was always hard to resist snacking on high-calorie foods. A lot of the foods served on the plane were rich and full of calories, and stopovers gave Terri the chance to eat in exotic restaurants.

Little by little, Terri began to notice she was putting on weight. She knew it was time to go on a diet, but doing two or three legs of cross-country trips a day didn't give her much time for finding, preparing, and eating diet foods. A stopover in San Juan or Mexico City also didn't give her the time to contemplate dieting.

One day, while on a flight to Honolulu, Terri met a passenger who had brought along the Fast Lane Diet Drink in a thermos. Terri had always been skeptical of "liquid" diets, but when she tasted the Diet Drink, she immediately asked for the recipe. It tasted just like a milk shake!

Terri couldn't wait to whip up a batch of the Diet Drink in her blender. Before long, she was concocting her own fruity recipes and sharing the drink with her roommates, who had ideas of their own for new drink recipes.

Terri loves the Fast Lane Fast because whenever she's 2, 3, or even 5 pounds overweight (particularly after a stopover in an exciting, romantic city), she can shed the excess weight in just thirty-six hours. Terri also uses the Fast Lane Diet Drink as life insurance—she knows she'll never truly let her weight get out of hand because the Diet Drink is always close at hand.

* * *

Type D Fast-Laner

NAME: Ron
AGE: 35
OCCUPATION: Art director

Back in art school, Ron had dreamed of becoming a big-city art director for a glossy magazine or maybe even a movie studio. He was a very talented student, who soon won awards for his inventive art direction. He moved to New York, where over the course of less than ten years he became the executive art director for a major women's magazine.

Life was very good to Ron. He traveled all over the world, directing photo sessions for covers and glamorous shots of models and celebrities for each issue. And all the while he was enjoying the perks of being art director on a magazine whose audience included the rich and the famous. But he was also enjoying a little too much of another good thing: the business lunch.

Recruiting stylists, models, and sponsors for his layouts was very much a part of Ron's business day. Ron began, at first without noticing it, to gain weight. His daily business lunch ritual was mandatory for business, so he felt trapped.

One day, over a business lunch with an art director from a competing magazine, Ron learned about the Business Lunch Diet, based on the Fast Lane Diet Drink. His friend showed him how he could eat a low-calorie meal in their favorite Italian restaurant, supplement it with the basic or flavored Fast Lane Diet Drink twice a day, and still lose weight.

Ron began to follow the Fast Lane Business Lunch Diet plan, sticking to low-calorie suggestions at his favorite business lunch restaurants. He brought the Diet Drink to work and had one at his desk for breakfast and one later in the evening for dinner. He was amazed at the rate at which he began to lose weight.

Now Ron, 20 pounds lighter, feels much better about himself. What truly amazes him is the way in which he was able to adjust his eating habits without making a change in his fast lane lifestyle.

Type E Fast-Laner

NAME: Joanne
AGE: Mid-forties
OCCUPATION: Real estate agent

Joanne was 32 when she married Jeff; by 44 she had filed for divorce. Although she had always enjoyed a vigorous social life and was an active member of her church, she was, in many ways, at loose ends. She had tried several careers: first teaching, then interior decorating (some of her clients sent her on glamorous trips to places like Spain and Hawaii), and then real estate. Joanne had a history of being unable to settle down to anything for much of her adult life.

When her marriage to Jeff began to fall apart, she was starting yet another career as a real estate agent and was doing very well, handling only the very upper-bracket homes for the agency.

But Joanne was beginning to gain weight. Her eating habits began to change, and she began to seek food as an answer to her loneliness. Her unhappiness and frustration caused her to eat more and more out of emotional upset—and less and less out of real hunger.

She would start her day by skipping breakfast, then ordering a jelly donut or two at the office and wolfing it down with coffee. Often she'd ignore lunches and lunchtime, too, feeling self-righteous about not eating the noon meal. But without fail, by 1:30 or 2:00 p.m. Joanne would be eating yet another high-calorie snack—and yet another at 3 p.m. Since she was often out with clients, she would be too busy to stop for a sandwich or a salad, especially late in the day.

Once she was home, which was sometimes not until seven or eight o'clock at night, Joanne would continue her snacking until bedtime. Although she knew that her eating habits were terrible, that she was putting on weight, and that what she was doing was downright *unhealthy*, she couldn't face the loneliness of sitting down to a meal by herself and rarely had the time

49

either to seek out or to prepare a good, balanced, weighed-and-measured meal.

Then one day Joanne ran into Connie, an old friend who worked for another real estate agency across town. Connie looked like a million. She was a member of the Million-Dollar Real Estate Sales Society and one of the top representatives in her corporation. Joanne just *had* to know what Connie was doing (other than being outrageously successful) that made her look so fabulous and so self-confident.

Connie told Joanne about the Fast Lane Diet Drink. She said it was like eating a milk shake three times a day. Not only that. She had a list of low-calorie snack foods that supplemented the Diet Drink; she could choose four low-calorie snacks a day.

Joanne loved the idea of the On-the-Road Diet. Not only did the concept fit in with her favorite way to eat but it also made sense in terms of the schedule she was on. She was already eating this way—just eating too much and the wrong kinds of foods—foods that were laden with empty calories.

The Diet Drink would also fit right in with her lifestyle because it took virtually no time to prepare and could be carried along with her—even in the car.

Joanne has been a real success—in her job and with her diet. Never once has she had to alter her fast lane lifestyle to slim down and look the part of a successful (and very attractive) single woman.

Type F Fast-Laner

Charlie, Chris, Ron, Terri, and Joanne. Each of them found a diet that *worked*, then switched over to the Staying-on-Course Diet, which helped each of them make the transition to a healthy eating pattern.

So, in a way, *every* Fast Lane dieter becomes a type F—but only after he or she has used one of the other diets successfully.

But what if you're now at a weight that's fairly comfortable for you, and you're looking for a two-week program you can use from time to time—whenever you want to get back in control?

Here's a profile of two type F's who do just that:

NAMES: Debra and Blake
AGES: 35 (each)
OCCUPATIONS: Interior designer and attorney

Debra and her husband Blake struck most people as the ideal couple. They were two really popular kids who fell in love, and they married right out of college. Debra immediately embarked upon her career as an interior designer, while Blake went on to law school. By the age of 30, both were successfully launched. And both were true fast-laners.

Debra found that she was on the run constantly and would grab something to eat whenever she could. Like most fast-laners, she had difficulty keeping tabs on her weight and really didn't notice she had added some extra pounds until she was weighed at her doctor's during a physical exam. She had always been proud of her figure and really resented the 10 extra pounds. So she began really thinking about what she was putting into her body and made a concentrated effort to change her eating habits. She started serving herself and Blake fewer red meat dishes—both were surprised at how much better they felt.

Then one day a colleague told Blake about the Fast Lane Diet Drink. It really appealed to both Debra and Blake because it was portable—something they could use for life. At this point neither of them needed to lose weight, but found that the two-week Staying-on-Course Diet helped them maintain their ideal weight.

Debra and Blake treat the Staying-on-Course Diet like a two-week vacation, two or three times a year. It gets both of them back on track, makes them aware of the food they're eating, and keeps them at a comfortable weight. Most importantly—especially to two busy fast-laners—it makes them feel wonderfully in control of their eating, so that weight gain is one less thing they have to think about.

THE SIX FAST LANE DIET PLANS

Now, go for it! Remember, if your lifestyle changes, feel free to try a different diet.

Before you begin, realize that no matter which plan you're on, you may supplement your diet with any quantity of the following beverages:

Seltzer water

Club soda*

Carbonated spring water

Diet soda*

Coffee†

Decaffeinated coffee

Tea†

*There is sodium in club soda and diet soda, so if you're on a salt-restricted diet, stay away.

†If you're already in the fast lane of life, the caffeine in coffee and tea is probably unnecessary and unhealthy. Watch how much you drink of these two beverages and try decaffeinated coffee or herbal tea as alternatives.

A Fast Lane Reality

For millions of fast-laners: If you must have an alcoholic drink, for whatever reason, here is the official Fast Lane Cocktail:

In a tall glass:

1 ounce of dry white wine

Crushed ice or several ice cubes

Seltzer or carbonated spring or mineral water

A twist of lemon or lime

This drink is called a wine spritzer. If it's the only non-fast lane thing you do all day, and you must imbibe booze, make yourself sip it slowly, and try to relax. If you need a chaser, have a plain glass of club soda or seltzer. Don't have more than one of these a day.

THE ORIGINAL FAST LANE DIET: For Type A Fast-Laners

The original Fast Lane Diet is a two-week program that features a varied menu in conjunction with the Fast Lane Diet Drink.

On this program *two* of your daily meals (breakfast and lunch *or* breakfast and dinner) consist of the Fast Lane Diet Drink (basic or flavored—the choice is yours). The third meal (lunch or dinner) will have approximately 400 calories, giving you from 840 to 1,000 calories per day, depending on which of the Fast Lane Diet Drinks you choose.

During this two-week program, you can expect to lose between 3 and 8 pounds in the first week and less in the second.

Here is the fourteen-day menu plan for the "third meal" of the day.

■ *First Day*

    1 cup hot instant bouillon*

    4 ounces broiled lean ground beef patty

---

*Those on a sodium-restricted diet may substitute a cup of hot or iced herb tea or homemade chicken soup, with all the fat skimmed off, for the hot instant bouillon.

½ cup cooked carrots, flavored with parsley and pepper

1 baked potato, topped with 2 tablespoons low-fat cottage cheese and dillweed (optional)

½ grapefruit

423 calories

■ **Second Day**

1 cup hot instant bouillon

4 ounces broiled cod with Butter Buds and pepper

1 cup broccoli with lemon juice to taste

1 baked potato with 2 tablespoons low-fat cottage cheese

1 slice dry whole wheat bread or toast

1 cup fresh or unsweetened frozen strawberries with 2 tablespoons low-fat yogurt

426 calories

■ **Third Day**

1 cup hot instant bouillon

1 broiled chicken breast, skin removed, with seasonings of your choice, chopped celery, and onion

1 cup rice cooked with seasonings of your choice, chopped celery, and onion

1 sliced tomato

1 orange, sliced and topped with chopped mint (optional)

424 calories

■ **Fourth Day**

1 cup hot instant bouillon

2-egg omelet made without butter and with ½ cup sliced mushrooms

Plenty of sliced tomatoes

1 slice dry whole wheat bread

½ cantaloupe, topped with 1 tablespoon low-fat yogurt and chopped mint (optional)

282 calories

■ **Fifth Day**

1 cup hot instant bouillon

1 roasted breast of chicken, skin removed

1 baked potato, topped with 2 tablespoons low-fat cottage cheese and chopped onion

1 cup green beans, cooked and topped with 1 tablespoon Parmesan cheese (optional)

Plenty of celery stalks

½ grapefruit

430 calories

■ **Sixth Day**

1 cup hot instant bouillon

4 ounces broiled flounder or any other lean, white-fleshed fish with lemon slice (optional)

1 medium boiled potato, topped with chopped parsley and chopped onion

1 cup mixed raw vegetable salad, tossed with 2 tablespoons low-calorie Italian dressing

½ bagel, no butter

½ cup fresh or frozen berries (any kind)

approximately 410 calories

■ **Seventh Day**

1 cup hot instant bouillon

1 baked potato, topped with ½ cup low-fat cottage cheese, chopped green pepper, and 2 tablespoons shredded cheddar cheese (melted under the broiler)

2 whole raw carrots

½ bagel, no butter

1 sliced peach with a sprinkling of cinnamon

421 calories

■ **Eighth Day**

1 cup hot instant bouillon

4 ounces roast turkey, skin removed

1 tablespoon cranberry-orange relish

1 salad, made of lettuce, 1 tablespoon sliced almonds, 1 sliced orange, 1 green onion, and sliced celery and topped with 2 tablespoons low-calorie Italian dressing or oil and vinegar

1 slice whole wheat bread or toast

441 calories

■ **Ninth Day**

1 cup hot instant bouillon

4 ounces broiled sliced flank steak with 1 tablespoon Worcestershire sauce (optional)

About 1 cup shredded cabbage with 1 tablespoon diet mayonnaise and caraway seeds

½ bagel, no butter

½ cantaloupe with fresh lime or lemon juice

415 calories

■ **Tenth Day**

1 cup hot instant bouillon

4 ounces baked flounder or other lean, white-fleshed fish served with sliced lemon and 1 tablespoon sliced almonds

½ cup cooked carrots, topped with 2 tablespoons cheddar cheese, 1 tablespoon chopped onion, and chopped dill

1 small bran muffin, no butter

½ cup any flavor Jell-O with low-fat topping

345 calories

■ **Eleventh Day**

1 cup hot instant bouillon

½ cup spinach or whole wheat noodles, cooked and topped with 2 tablespoons grated Parmesan cheese, chopped parsley, chopped celery, 1 tablespoon diced onion, and ½ cup raw mushrooms and seasoned with pepper and garlic

½ cup low-fat cottage cheese on lettuce with a handful of sliced radishes

½ grapefruit, heated under broiler and garnished with chopped mint

317 calories

■ **Twelfth Day**

1 cup hot instant bouillon

1 tuna salad, made with a 6½-ounce can water-packed tuna, 1 hard-boiled egg, 1 tablespoon diet mayonnaise, sliced celery, ¼ cup chopped onion, and garlic and lemon juice to taste

1 salad, made with one carrot and a handful of cucumbers, green peppers, radishes, and zucchini

416 calories

■ **Thirteenth Day**

1 cup hot instant bouillon

4 ounces bay scallops, broiled, or sautéed in 1 tablespoon diet margarine and seasoned with paprika and lemon juice and sprinkled with chopped parsley

1 cup sliced carrots, raw or cooked, with chopped dill

1 slice rye bread, plain or toasted, no butter

½ cantaloupe or other seasonal fresh fruit

337 calories

* * *

■ *Fourteenth Day*

1 cup canned Manhattan clam chowder plus ¼ ounce canned clams plus 1 cup skim milk*

10 oyster crackers

1 salad of spinach leaves with plenty of sliced raw, fresh mushrooms, 1 tablespoon unsalted sunflower seeds, 1 tablespoon raisins, and 2 tablespoons low-calorie Italian dressing

½ cup fresh or unsweetened frozen berries

425 calories

*Those on a sodium-restricted diet may substitute the following for the clam chowder:
1 cup pasta shells cooked *al dente* and served cold, mixed with ½ cup low-fat cottage cheese, chopped parsley, and pepper and garlic to taste (*190 calories*).

8

THE PASSING LANE
DIET: For Type B
Fast-Laners

On this two-week diet plan two of your daily meals will consist of the Fast Lane Diet Drink (have it for breakfast and dinner or for breakfast and lunch, whichever suits your day's schedule).

Your third meal of the day (lunch or dinner) is a fast lane fast food—you may choose among frozen entrées, canned or prepared dinners, or food from a fast-food restaurant. The choice is yours. Whatever you choose, you vow not to eat *more than 400 calories per meal.*

Plus—and for those in the Passing Lane this is most important—you hardly have to do a thing! No meal preparation. No food weighing. Very little shopping.

Before you get in the passing lane:

- The Passing Lane Diet offers a fourteen-day menu. This menu is provided for your convenience, but if you have difficulty finding any of the items on the menu, you may substitute by using foods from the appendix, which lists fast foods and their calorie counts.

- Since the Passing Lane Diet doesn't provide the dieter with a lot of fiber, I recommend that *at least* one of the daily Fast Lane Diet drinks be a fruity variation. If, however, you prefer the basic Diet Drink, I suggest you add a piece of fruit from the following list to your daily menu:

  1 medium nectarine
  1 medium peach
  2 plums
  1 cup watermelon (2 generous slices)
  1 Bosc pear
  1 medium orange
  1 cup fresh or frozen unsweetened berries
  1 banana

- **First Day** (lunch or dinner)

  1 Hardee's cheeseburger, Burger King Whopper, Jr., or McDonald's cheeseburger with standard condiments

  or

  2 White Castle cheeseburgers

  or

  1 Stouffer's frozen beef Stroganoff dinner

- **Second Day** (lunch or dinner)

  1 Taco Bell bean burrito

  or

  1 Green Giant boil-in-bag sloppy Joe with 1 hamburger bun

  or

  1 serving Buitoni lasagne with meat sauce

- **Third Day** (lunch or dinner)

  2 pieces Arthur Treacher's fish with lemon slices

  or

  1 11-ounce Van de Kamp's frozen fish fillet

  or

  ½ package Swanson fish and chips

- **Fourth Day** (lunch or dinner)

    1 5-ounce Arby's roast beef sandwich

    or

    1 Morton's beef enchilada (12-ounce package)

    or

    1 Banquet beef pot pie

- **Fifth Day** (lunch or dinner)

    2 slices standard, thin-sliced Pizza Hut cheese pizza

    or

    1 Weight Watchers frozen 6-ounce cheese pizza

    or

    1 Stouffer's French bread pizza (half of 10¼-ounce package)

- **Sixth Day** (lunch or dinner)

    1 serving Weight Watchers frozen chicken oriental

    or

    1 piece Church's fried chicken

    or

    1 Stouffer's frozen chicken à la king

- **Seventh Day** (lunch or dinner)

    1 11-ounce frozen La Choy Chinese chicken dinner

    or

    1 Chun King chicken or shrimp chow mein frozen dinner

    or

    1 package Arthur Treacher's shrimp

- **Eighth Day** (lunch or dinner)

    1 Dairy Queen chili dog

    or

2 Taco Bell beef tacos

or

1 Swanson macaroni and cheese dinner

■ **Ninth Day** (lunch or dinner)

2 White Castle fish sandwiches

or

1 9-ounce package Taste-o-Sea fried flounder

or

1 Stouffer's tuna noodle frozen casserole

■ **Tenth Day** (lunch or dinner)

1 Arby's 5½-ounce ham and cheese sandwich

or

1 Golden cheese blintz with 2 tablespoons sour cream

or

1 package Mrs. Paul's frozen eggplant Parmesan

■ **Eleventh Day** (lunch or dinner)

1 10½-ounce container Stouffer's frozen lasagne

or

1 15-ounce can Buitoni cheese ravioli

or

1 Burger King Whopper, Jr.

■ **Twelfth Day** (lunch or dinner)

1 15-ounce can Buitoni spaghetti and meatballs

or

1 13-ounce package Weight Watchers lasagne with cheese, veal, and sauce

or

1 package Green Giant veal parmigiana (7-ounce baked entrée)

■ **Thirteenth Day** (lunch or dinner)

1 Gino's Sirloiner

or

1 salad bar salad made with lettuce, bean sprouts, cucumber, radishes, green peppers, 1 tablespoon grated cheese, and 1 teaspoon bacon bits with 1 tablespoon Italian, French, or Russian dressing

or

1 8¾-ounce can Heinz franks and beans in tomato sauce

■ **Fourteenth Day** (lunch or dinner)

1 can Hormel chili without beans

or

1 portion Wendy's chili plus small salad bar salad made with mixed greens, cucumber, radishes, 1 tablespoon shredded cheese, and 1 tablespoon diet dressing

or

1 Stouffer's beef teriyaki with rice and vegetables

9

THE FAST LANE FAST:
For Type C Fast-Laners

It's easy to use the Fast Lane Fast. All you do is drink the Fast Lane Diet Drink *four* times a day for three days.

Have it during meal times—perhaps one for breakfast, one for lunch, one as an afternoon snack, and one for dinner. Or have your fourth drink before bedtime instead of in the afternoon.

I also recommend that *at least two* of your Fast Lane Diet Drinks be fruity versions. If you prefer the basic Diet Drink, you may supplement the Fast Lane Fast with two pieces of fruit daily from the list on page 62.

After three days, go back to a moderate pattern of eating, or spend two weeks on the Staying-on-Course Diet (type F), and you will look better, feel better, and be ready for whichever fast track you're on.

A word of caution.   I do not recommend that you stay on the Fast Lane Fast for longer than three days. It is a good idea to check with your doctor before going on *any* diet.

Before you get started on your Fast Lane Fast, here are some interesting facts about fasting:

When your fast ends, you usually find that meat is less desirable to you.

With fasting, you control your body rather than having it control you. And fast-laners like to be in control.

When you go on the Fast Lane Fast, you will be amazed that you are not hungry.

Some people claim that fasting makes them feel cleansed, renewed, and more energetic.

The Fast Lane Fast may or may not increase your energy level. It will certainly take off weight and it's the safest, easiest, least time-consuming way of doing so that I know about. If it also gives you a boost, consider it a much-needed bonus. Fast-laners need all the vitality they can get.

10

THE BUSINESS LUNCH DIET:
For Type D Fast-Laners

The Business Lunch Diet provides you with a business lunch or dinner meal that is low in calories (no more than 500 calories) and can be found in a variety of business lunch restaurants.

I have purposely used some of the more common dishes from each kind of cuisine: French, Italian, Chinese, Japanese, Mexican, and deli. An exotic dish or two might be perfect for the Fast Lane Diet but might not be found in very many restaurants. What I've tried to give the business-luncher is a varied menu that can be ordered just about anywhere.

The business meal will be supplemented by having the Fast Lane Diet Drink in the flavor of your choice for two meals a day. If you need to have a business lunch, have the Diet Drink for breakfast and dinner. Of course, if your business is over dinner rather than lunch, you may switch your "business lunch diet" and make it your "business dinner diet."*

Before you begin, here are some pointers all business-lunchers should note:

- Most restaurants cater to the appetite of a 200-pound man. In most cases, you'll be better off eating about *half* the portion that's served to you.

---

*Exact calorie counts are impossible for foods eaten out, but I've included calorie counts for *average*-sized portions in the appendix. Be moderate!

- It's a good idea always to begin your business lunch or dinner by eating the *least caloric* food first. If you're served a vegetable along with your entrée, eat the vegetable first.

- Order a glass of club soda, seltzer, tea, coffee, or diet soda and drink it before your food arrives. This will help curb your appetite for some of the more tempting, high-calorie foods to come.

- If your dining partner doesn't object, have the bread and butter removed from the table—better yet, ask that it not be brought to the table. Most of us find it nearly impossible to resist warm bread, especially in a French or Italian restaurant.

Recipes are provided in Chapter 13 for all asterisked dishes mentioned in this chapter.

Go Signs in the Fast Lane, Italian Style

Here is my suggestion for your Italian business lunch—a menu that can be ordered in nearly any Italian restaurant you (or they) choose:

Carbonated mineral water with lemon or lime wedge

Stracciatella (chicken broth with beaten egg)*

Insalata mista (mixed greens with tomato wedges served with lemon wedges and red wine vinegar)

Pesce de giorno (fish of the day, poached or grilled)

or

Mussels marinara (mussels steamed in white wine)

Fresh fruit served without cream or sugar

Some other low-calorie suggestions for the Italian business lunch:

Vegetable antipasto (as a main dish meal, without oil)

Prosciutto con melone (ham and cantaloupe)

Linguine alle vongole (linguine with white clam sauce)

Sorgiano (swordfish, marinated and broiled)

Veal paillard or chop (without breading)

Stop Signs for the Italian Business Lunch

Don't eat the delicious but dangerous Italian hard rolls with butter or the tempting garlic bread. The roll alone contains over 200 calories!

A good Italian restaurant prepares food to order, so don't be afraid to order it *exactly as you want it*—without cream, broiled instead of sautéed, with half the usual amount of cheese, and so on. Remember that most good chefs are anxious to please.

To season your food, use fresh lemon juice instead of butter and salt.

For pasta lovers

Pasta itself is not terribly high in calories, but the sauces put on pasta *are*.

Try limiting or doing without high-calorie sauces and make the complex carbohydrates found in the pasta fuel you for the rest of your fast lane business day. Parmesan cheese, in moderation, is an excellent topping for pasta.

Cold pasta is delicious and tastes great without rich sauces. Try cold linguine mixed with broccoli and lemon juice. It's fabulous. Remember: Whatever you dream up, the chef can probably prepare.

If you *love* spaghetti and meatballs, do without the meatballs. They can be over 150 calories apiece!

Limit your pasta intake to about a cup and a half.

Go Signs in the Fast Lane, French Style

Nouvelle cuisine ("new cooking") is very "in" now in French dining, and that means a lot of French dishes utilizing fresh fruits and vegetables and fewer of the richer sauces and large portions French food was once so famous for.

In addition, *nouvelle cuisine* uses a lot of seafood and poultry—two mainstays of a fast-laner's business lunch.

Remember: In a good French restaurant the food is cooked *à la minute* (to order), and you can expect to have your food prepared exactly the way you want to eat it. Ask your waiter to prepare your favorite dish without the cream, sautéed in *half* the usual amount of butter, or in any way you wish. In a good restaurant there is enough talent in the kitchen to do anything you ask the staff to do.

Here is the menu for your Fast Lane Business Lunch, French style:

Carbonated mineral water with a lemon or lime wedge

Huîtres fraîches (fresh oysters on the half shell)

or

A cup of beef consommé

and

Salade Niçoise (tuna with a mixture of greens and vegetables—ask them to omit the anchovies)

or

Braised filet of lemon sole

Fruits frais et sorbet (seasonal fruits and sorbet made of the same fruit)

Here are some other low-calorie suggestions for the French business lunch:

Small portion celeri rémoulade (celery root salad)

2-egg omelet with caviar

Entrecôte aux trois poivres (loin cut of beef cooked with three different peppers)

Grilled chicken (with garlic and seasoning to taste)

Braised artichoke provençal (a delicious, time-consuming treat: not for your busiest day of the year)

Santé potage. In France almost any restaurant will have this soup on the menu. It's almost thought of as a spring health tonic. It is very low in calories, contains sorrel leaves, and is quite delicious. I've included a recipe for this tasty soup in Chapter 13.

Stop Signs for the French Business Lunch

When ordering vegetables, ask to have them steamed or boiled rather than sautéed.

Always order à la carte in a French restaurant to make certain you don't get a lot of tempting but nondietetic garnishes.

The french bread in a French restaurant is *absolutely forbidden* to dieters! Steer very clear.

Avoid hollandaise sauce, which contains 170 calories for only one-half cup. In fact, avoid *most* French sauces. If you do order them, make certain they are brought to the table "on the side."

Go Signs in the Fast Lane, Chinese Style

Don't make the mistake of many business-lunchers. I've overheard fast-laners saying, "Let's go for Chinese. It's not fattening." Then they zero in on some of the richer, saucier Chinese foods, laden with black bean sauce, lobster sauce, sweet and sour sauce—and their low-calorie meal turns into a dieter's disaster.

It's so easy to avoid this because Chinese cuisine is basically excellent for fast-laners. It is rich in vegetables, such as water chestnuts, snow peas, bamboo shoots, Chinese cabbage—all good sources of vitamins and minerals and all low in calories.

One of my favorite things about eating in Chinese restaurants is that they are light on desserts. Usually, only fresh fruit is served; I'm generally happy with my soothing cup of Chinese tea.

* * *

Suggested menu for your Chinese Business Lunch:

1 cup egg drop soup

or

1 cup hot and sour soup

and

1 portion chicken with water chestnuts *without noodles or rice*

or

1 portion scallops with vegetables *without noodles* on ½ cup white rice

or

1 order moo goo gai pan

and

Fresh fruit or 1 fortune cookie with hot tea

Other low-calorie suggestions for the Chinese business lunch:

1 cup sesame chicken salad

1½ cups chicken with litchis

1 portion long soup (pork strips and vegetables in broth)

1 portion chicken chow mein with ½ cup noodles and ½ cup rice

Stop Signs for the Chinese Business Lunch

Chinese cuisine relies heavily on stir frying. When ordering your meal in a Chinese restaurant, request that your selection be sautéed in chicken broth instead of oil.

Some Chinese appetizers sound more dietetic than they are: Do not even *consider* ordering shrimp toast, foil chicken, chicken in paper, or shrimp balls. They are too high in calories for the amount of food you get.

Soy sauce is usually on the table in Chinese restaurants; try not to use it. It's extremely high in sodium, which is bad for your health and causes water retention, which will impair weight loss. If you must add something to your food, go for the mustard! It's low in calories and great with most Chinese dishes, but it is *very hot.*

Happily, there's no bread on the table—but beware the fried Chinese noodles. A tablespoon won't kill you, but have you ever been able to stop at one tablespoon? If you're waiting for your food to arrive and feeling ravenous, try sipping some Chinese tea instead.

Go Signs in the Fast Lane, Japanese Style

Most Japanese food is ideal for fast lane dieters because it is generally low in calories. Maybe that's why the Japanese business lunch is increasing in popularity. One New York friend told me she eats Japanese food three times a week. Sushi bars are springing up everywhere. Sushi is raw fish with rice that has been shaped, cured, and arranged in very special ways. It tastes fantastic and is naturally low in calories.

The delicious, clear soups that are standard with most Japanese meals are another plus. If you're a fast lane dieter, take advantage of these naturally low-calorie and delicious filler-uppers.

Here is the menu for the fast-laner's Japanese business lunch diet:

> 1 cup miso soup with bean curd *or* clear soup with fish balls
> *and*
> 1 portion Japanese cucumber salad *or* Japanese lettuce and seaweed salad
> *or*
> Oshinko (pickled vegetables)
> *and*
> 1 portion sashimi, assorted (raw fish)
> *or*

1 portion teppan-yaki (sliced beef steak grilled with vegetables)
and

Tea, hot or cold, or black coffee

Here are some other low-calorie suggestions for the Japanese business lunch:

Shabu-shabu (beef and vegetables in broth)·

Yosenabe (fish stew)

Miso soup with Chinese cabbage

Spinach, fish, and tofu steamed in sake

Nimono (steamed vegetables and minced chicken)

Chicken yakitori (chicken on skewers)

Beef sukiyaki (beef and vegetables)

Stop Signs for the Japanese Business Lunch

Not *all* Japanese foods are low in calories. Tempura, prepared with a batter-fried coating, is a poor choice for dieters!

Soy sauce (shoyu) is used plentifully in Japanese cooking, so avoid Japanese cuisine entirely if you are watching your salt intake.

Japanese desserts can be deceiving. Stay away from ice cream, deep-fried fruit, candied chestnuts, and strawberries in snow. All are high in calories.

Go Signs in the Fast Lane down Mexico Way

The truth about Mexican food may surprise you. Mexican food, when ordered judiciously, can actually be low in calories.

I go to Mexican restaurants in the summer because I love gazpacho, a fabulous tomato-and-cucumber-based soup with onions and plenty of spices. It's served cold, and if you ask your waiter for a double portion, you can make it your meal—a very filling and low-calorie one.

I also love tacos, and I've learned that if I order them with shrimp or vegetable fillings instead of meat, I cut way back on the calories. And besides, they're a great change of pace.

Here is the menu for the Fast Lane Mexican business lunch:

Carbonated spring water with a twist of lemon or lime or iced tea, diet soda, or coffee

and

4 plain nacho chips with no more than 1 tablespoon of guacamole dip

and

Pollo en salsa verde (chicken with green sauce)—no rice or beans

or

1 huevo ranchero (egg with spicy sauce)

and

Mexican coffee (flavored with cinnamon)

Some other low-calorie suggestions for a Mexican business lunch:

Tortilla soup (one bowl only—and make it a complete lunch)

Shrimp taco

Shredded chicken taco

Taco salad without sour cream or guacamole

Stop Signs for a Mexican Business Lunch

Go easy on the kidney beans—they're over 200 calories per cup, which is fine, if that's all you eat. Ditto for refried beans—sorry, folks.

An 8-ounce margarita is a fast lane downer at 348 calories.

If you're served an otherwise fast-laner's diet selection, but it's garnished with sour cream or cheese topping or both, get rid of the garnish and you'll save more than 100 calories.

When in doubt, always order vegetable fillings instead of meat.

Go Signs in the Fast Lane, Deli Style

If you have business lunches in New York or in one of America's larger cosmopolitan cities, you know that many a meeting takes place over an overstuffed corned beef sandwich.

The trademark of a deli meal is the dill, sour, or kosher pickle. And that's good news because kosher dills are low in calorie. One bit of bad news for the sodium-conscious: They are high in salt, so beware.

But what about other deli favorites? Obviously, overstuffed sandwiches are taboo, but you can still enjoy your favorite deli meats if they're lean cuts and you eat them without the bread.

Chopped chicken liver, believe it or not, is safe for fast lane dieters—providing you eat only half a cup. And you'll still have room left for half a cup of sliced cucumbers in vinegar.

And if you absolutely can't live without your bottle of Dr. Brown's Cel-Ray Tonic or Cream Soda, there's good news: The good doctor now makes both old standbys in diet versions.

There are plenty of other good bets at the deli. Here's a menu I think all fast lane deli dieters will enjoy:

1 Dr. Brown's Diet Cel-Ray tonic *or* Dr. Brown's diet cream soda. Or you may substitute carbonated spring water, coffee, or tea

and

1 bagel with lox and cream cheese (limit yourself to no more than 2 slices of lox)

or

2 cheese blintzes with a tablespoon of sour cream

or

2 medium pieces of gefilte fish with 1 tablespoon white horseradish *and* 1 slice rye bread without butter

and

1 large sour pickle

Some other low-calorie suggestions for the fast lane deli dieter:

- 1 portion cold borscht without sour cream topping (as your main course)
- A 2-egg onion omelet with one slice dry whole wheat toast
- 1 tuna salad sandwich on rye bread (make sure it is water-packed tuna)
- 1 bowl chicken matzoh ball soup with 2 crackers

Stop Signs for the Deli Business Lunch

Cole slaw can be OK as long as you don't eat more than a heaping tablespoon.

Deli corned beef and pastrami, when ultralean, can be OK if consumed in small (2-ounce) quantities without bread. But most of the time these deli delicacies are very fatty and can slow down anyone in the fast lane.

Don't order any sandwiches or hot dishes that are cooked with chicken fat. Most delis announce when they use real chicken fat, so you needn't do much detective work.

Potato knishes—mmm, delicious—are very high in calories, so don't go for them *unless that's all you're planning to eat.* And then, you may have only one.

11

THE ON-THE-ROAD DIET: For Type E Fast-Laners

Snackers and grazers have the one thing fast-laners love and need most of all: *choice!* On the two-week On-the-Road Diet you get to choose from three food lists of delicious, healthful snacks of 100 calories or less. You choose *one snack from each of these three groups* daily.

You may also have a "bonus snack" from group four—the goodies list—or, if you prefer, you make take your bonus snack from one of the other three groups.

You will supplement this approximately 400-calories-per-day snacking menu with *two Fast Lane Diet Drinks per day*. These may be basic Fast Lane Diet Drinks or fruity variations. The choice is yours.

I recommend that you have one of the Fast Lane Diet Drinks in the morning as a breakfast energizer and one late in the afternoon or before bed. The snacks should be spread out over the course of the day—but, of course, this is the way snackers and grazers eat, so that should be second nature to you.

Here are some pointers for on-the-road dieters:

DON'T repeat a snack on the same day, but feel free to have a snack you particularly like once a day for each day you're on the diet.

DON'T take more than one snack from the goodies list, group four.

DON'T stay on the diet for more than two weeks. Follow it up with a sensible, moderate eating program like the Staying-on-Course Diet, type F.

DO supplement the On-the-Road Diet with a daily multivitamin tablet. (See Chapter 15 for tips on vitamins for fast-laners.)

■ *Group 1 Snacks*

2 cups popcorn, unbuttered and unsalted

3 Ritz crackers, 1 teaspoon cream cheese on each

1 medium oatmeal cookie

3 wheat thins, each spread with 1 teaspoon Snack-Mate cheese spread

2 Stella D'Oro egg biscuits

2 Stella D'Oro sesame breadsticks

2 Triscuit wafers, 1 teaspoon peanut butter on each

⅔ cup Wheat Chex cereal

2 graham crackers with 1 teaspoon grape jam on each

5 melba rounds with 1 teaspoon low-fat cottage cheese on each

½-inch slice Dromedary date nut roll with 1 teaspoon cream cheese

½ English muffin with 1 tablespoon jam

2 Fig Newtons fig cakes

1 plain croissant

½ bagel with 1 teaspoon butter or margarine

1 Pillsbury buttermilk biscuit with 1 tablespoon low-calorie jam

* * *

■ *Group 2 Snacks*

1 ounce Edam cheese

12 shelled whole almonds, unsalted

1 ounce farmer's cheese

1 4-ounce jar Sau-Sea shrimp cocktail

1 Lipton cream of chicken Cup-a-Soup

10 medium cashew nuts

1 hard-boiled egg

1 8-ounce container plain low-fat yogurt

1 slice American cheese

4 ¼-ounce sticks beef jerky

1 slice smoked turkey wrapped around 1 dill spear

2 slices cooked ham

2 Keebler sesame crackers, each spread with 1 teaspoon Brie cheese

1 ounce Swiss Knight or Borden's Gruyère cheese

1 frozen yogurt on a stick, uncoated

■ *Group 3 Snacks*

1 medium nectarine

1 Bosc pear

1 Granny Smith apple

2 cups diced watermelon

4–6 parboiled or raw broccoli spears dipped in 2 tablespoons sour cream

1 carrot, cut into sticks and dipped in 1 tablespoon of Dijon mustard

1 banana

1 large orange

1 ounce Sun Maid dried fruit bits

8 large dried apricots

1 cup fresh cherries

1 cup fresh pineapple

4 sticks celery stuffed with 3 tablespoons grated cheddar

1 cold, cooked artichoke dipped in 2 tablespoons sour cream

1 red or green bell pepper, sliced and dipped in 2 tablespoons low-fat yogurt

cucumber sandwiches (½ sliced cucumber with ½ tablespoon peanut butter *or* 1 tablespoon cream cheese)

■ *Group 4 Snacks (Optional)*

1 ounce Raisinets

1 ounce jelly beans

4 nacho cheese-flavored tortilla chips dipped in 1 tablespoon salsa

1 Sara Lee cinnamon roll

1 piece Drake's pound cake, plain or marble

1 Hostess plain, cinnamon, or powdered doughnut

½ cup Jell-O gelatin dessert

1 orange Creamsicle

1 ounce licorice (Switzer)

1 twin Popsicle

1 pretzel rod

2 Oreo cream filled cookies

1 scoop orange sherbet

12

THE STAYING-ON-COURSE DIET:
For Type F Fast-Laners

The Staying-on-Course Diet is a two-week transition diet designed to gradually increase your food intake and ease you into a healthier eating pattern. It offers two low-calorie meals per day, which you supplement with one Fast Lane Diet Drink, basic or flavored, and a daily multivitamin.

That's all there is to it.

Of course, as an anxious fast-laner, you might want to know why. If you're feeling good about your weight right now and you're into a healthier way of life, why not just get right back into the swing of things?

You see, statistics show that most dieters are likely to gain back most of the weight they lose—*within two weeks of going off a diet!* To make matters worse, each time you go on a diet, the weight is harder and harder to lose. Why?

It's really very simple. When you go on a diet, your body takes in less food. But the body stores food as fat; it burns its fat supply at a set rate, called your basal metabolism. When you diet, your body lowers its basal metabolism and begins burning the supplies more slowly. When you go off the diet, your body doesn't know it immediately and continues to burn calories at the slower rate. What this all means is that even if you eat the same food you ate before you went on the diet, your body won't be burning it as efficiently. So you're likely to gain back the weight you've lost—and may even gain back more.

A "transition" diet like the Staying-on-Course Diet prevents this from happening because when you *gradually* increase your food intake, your body has a fighting chance to get back on course.

You also have a new friend traveling with you in the fast lane: the Fast Lane Diet Drink. Even after your two weeks on the Staying-on-Course Diet, you can and should make the Fast Lane Diet Drink *a part of your daily life.* Use it as a third meal, a between-meal snack-on-the-run, or—if you find yourself putting on a pound or two—try using the Fast Lane Fast (see p. 67) for thirty-six hours of quick weight loss.

The Staying-on-Course Diet is really nothing more than a sensible daily eating plan together with a portable dietary supplement—the Diet Drink. I think you will be amazed at how easily it conforms to your fast lane lifestyle.

The Staying-on-Course Diet

■ *Breakfast* (same every day)

½ grapefruit *or* ½ cup fresh fruit *or* ½ apple

1 slice toasted whole wheat bread

1 tablespoon butter

Coffee or tea, black

210 calories

■ *Lunch or Dinner* (same every day)

1 cup Diet Drink* with 1 slice whole wheat bread or toast with 1 tablespoon butter

*Calorie count depends on Diet Drink selection. See Chapter 3.

■ *Lunch or Dinner, Day One*

1½ cups spaghetti with mushroom or meat sauce*

1 large vegetable salad with 2 tablespoons diet dressing

Fresh fruit for dessert

about 450 calories

*Stouffer's Lean Cuisine spaghetti and meat sauce has 300 calories and is very good.

■ *Lunch or Dinner, Day Two*

4 ounces broiled steak (fat removed)

1 baked potato with 1 tablespoon butter or margarine

Mushrooms sautéed in bouillon* or broiled

1 cup fresh, canned, or frozen broccoli sprinkled with
   1 tablespoon Parmesan cheese

½ cup flavored diet gelatin for dessert

542 calories

*Do not use bouillon if on a sodium-restricted diet.

■ *Lunch or Dinner, Day Three*

1 broiled breast of chicken with skin and fat removed

1 cup cooked noodles with 1 tablespoon Parmesan cheese

1 large vegetable salad with 1 tablespoon diet dressing

2 Stella D'Oro biscuits

436 calories

■ *Lunch or Dinner, Day Four*

4 ounces broiled flounder or any other lean, white-fleshed fish
   with a dash of lemon juice, garlic, and lemon pepper
   seasoning

½ baked acorn squash with 1 teaspoon butter or margarine,
   dash of nutmeg

1 large mixed raw vegetable salad with 1 tablespoon diet dressing

½ cup flavored diet gelatin with diet or fresh cherries

325 calories

■ **Lunch or Dinner, Day Five**

4 ounces broiled lean hamburger with slice of raw onion (optional)

1 baked tomato sprinkled with basil and 1 tablespoon breadcrumbs

½ cup rainbow sherbet

547 calories

■ **Lunch or Dinner, Day Six**

4 ounces red snapper or scallops or any lean, white-fleshed fish, broiled with lemon juice and pepper

½ cup egg noodles with 1 tablespoon Parmesan cheese, ½ teaspoon of capers, and 1 tablespoon butter

1 cup cooked green beans and carrots, flavored with a pinch of dill

Blueberries in ¼ cup skim milk

475 calories

■ **Lunch or Dinner, Day Seven**

Tuna and noodle casserole*

Large vegetable salad with 1 tablespoon diet dressing

1 cup frozen unsweetened raspberries with 1 teaspoon ricotta cheese

580 calories

*Stouffer's tuna noodle casserole has 400 calories and is delicious.

* * *

Lunch or Dinner, Day Eight

Oriental beef with vegetables and rice*

Large vegetable salad with 1 tablespoon diet dressing

½ cup flavored diet gelatin or 1 piece fresh fruit

460 calories

*Stouffer's Lean Cuisine oriental beef with vegetables and rice has 300 cal-ories. If you stir-fry your own, use about 4 ounces of flank steak marinated in 3 tablespoons teriyaki sauce.

■ Lunch or Dinner, Day Nine

1 16-ounce Cornish hen, fat and skin removed (basted with diet grapefruit soda or diet ginger ale)

½ cup wild rice with mushrooms

1 cup cooked green beans flavored with a pinch of dill

½ cup orange sections sprinkled with chopped mint leaves (1 orange)

460 calories

■ Lunch or Dinner, Day Ten

8 ounces raw shrimp, peeled and deveined, sautéed in 1 teaspoon lime juice and ½ teaspoon vegetable oil

½ cup brown rice

1 cup cooked spinach mixed with 1 tablespoon plain yogurt and seasoned with garlic powder

1 sliced peach

434 calories

■ Lunch or Dinner, Day Eleven

1 large chicken salad made with 1 chicken breast, 1 tablespoon almonds, ¼ cup pineapple chunks, and 2 tablespoons diet mayonnaise, served on lettuce

½ bagel with 1 teaspoon butter or diet margarine

½ cup flavored diet gelatin

449 calories

■ *Lunch or Dinner, Day Twelve*

1 portion eggplant parmigiana*

1 tossed green salad made with lettuce, cherry tomatoes, chopped onion, green pepper, and a dash of basil or oregano

1 baked apple with sprinkling of cinnamon and artificial sweetener

505 calories

*Weight Watchers eggplant parmigiana is 280 calories and very good.

■ *Lunch or Dinner, Day Thirteen*

4 ounces broiled flounder or other lean, white-fleshed fish with dash of lemon juice, garlic powder, sweet basil, and cracked peppercorns

½ cup noodles with 1 tablespoon Parmesan cheese

½ cup mushrooms sautéed in bouillon*

½ cup cooked broccoli with 1 tablespoon butter

½ cup whipped ricotta cheese with artificial sweetener to taste and a dash of cinnamon

460 calories

*Do not use bouillon if you are on a sodium-restricted diet.

■ *Lunch or Dinner, Day Fourteen*

2 broiled lamb chops

1 broiled tomato with 1 tablespoon Parmesan cheese, oregano, and garlic powder

1 baked potato

1 cup S&W fruit salad or fresh fruit salad composed of 3 grapefruit sections, 4 orange slices, 3 to 4 white grapes, and ¼ sliced banana

449 calories

13

FAST LANE RECIPES FOR FAST LANE COOKS

What about fast-laners who really do a lot of cooking? Do you find yourself rotating approximately ten recipes for those large family meals—Sunday dinners, holiday dinners, birthdays?

Many home economists and nutritionists state that most American families run their kitchens on ten basic recipes a year. If you're in the fast lane, you no doubt recognize this pattern. Who has time to dream up new ideas for dinner? You probably prefer recipes that are fast and easy; you have no time to experiment. And tried-and-true recipes are familiar to the family; other family members can help prepare them, thus cutting down on preparation time.

But if you are following one of the Fast Lane Diets, you're now more aware of cutting those empty calories. So, with your newfound knowledge, take a look at your "basic ten" recipes and see how they might be modified. Can you cut some of the fats? Use less salt? Use leaner meats? Or should your "basic ten" be discarded altogether in favor of new low-calorie menus?

Here are some fast lane recipes straight from my own fast lane kitchen. They are absolutely delicious and easy to prepare. Perhaps you'll want to adapt them to your own fast lane lifestyle.

■ **Cedric Adams Casserole**

Cedric Adams was a popular WCCO radio personality in the Twin Cities. He always had a weight problem and was constantly looking for ways to shed pounds. He gave this favorite recipe to his listening public. I make it almost every week.

1 pound very lean ground beef

1 medium chopped onion

1 cup chopped celery

½ head chopped cabbage

1 can condensed tomato soup

Brown beef, onion, and celery in a nonstick pan. Drain fat as it accumulates. In a 1-quart casserole, alternate layers of ground beef mixture with the chopped cabbage. Pour on tomato soup (undiluted). Cover and bake at 350°F for about 1 hour.

Serves four

280 calories per serving

■ **Chicken Breasts Dijon**

This recipe was given to me by a good friend. It's super-easy, nutritious, tasty, and very low-calorie—and, best of all, it takes no time to prepare. My whole family loves it!

Boned chicken breasts (as many as the number of people you are serving)

Dijon mustard (1 teaspoon per chicken breast)

Remove any chicken fat and skin. Pound chicken flat with mallet. Lay breasts on lightly greased, nonstick pan. Spread 1 teaspoon mustard on each breast and bake at 350°F for 20 minutes.

180 calories per serving

■ **Light but Terrific Open-Face Tuna Rolls**

Here's a real fast lane family recipe we've used forever! It's economical, low-calorie, and easy enough for a 5-year-old to prepare. I've served this many times for dinner along with a big salad or a hot bowl of soup.

1 6½-ounce can water-packed tuna fish

Dijon mustard

4 slices low-calorie American or cheddar cheese

1 sliced cucumber

2 whole wheat hamburger buns

On each half of a hamburger bun, spread 1 teaspoon of mustard. Layer each with ¼ can tuna and with cucumber slices. Cover with 1 slice cheese and pop under broiler. Broil until cheese is melted.

Serves four

170 calories per serving

■ Baked Fish à la Fast Lane

This is a neighborhood favorite and has been used at more gatherings than I can count. We use orange roughy, a fish that's in great supply in Minnesota. But any lean, white-fleshed fish will do. If you don't have fresh fish, use frozen, unbreaded fish fillets.

6 white fish fillets

1 package frozen spinach souffle, thawed

Parmesan cheese, to taste

Spread fish on a flat, nonstick pan. Cover with the defrosted spinach souffle. Sprinkle with Parmesan cheese and bake at 350°F for no more than 30 minutes.

Makes six servings

180 calories per serving

■ Simple Salmon for a Crowd

Salmon is incredibly delicious, but it is a bit expensive. We have a relative on the West Coast who often sends us a salmon. Here's what we do with it:

½ whole salmon

1 cup mayonnaise*

---

*At times of stricter weight control, substitute low-calorie mayonnaise.

■ *Simple Salmon for a Crowd* (continued)

"Slather" mayonnaise on salmon—inside and out. Place on non-stick pan and bake at 350°F for 30 minutes. Cool. Then refrigerate overnight.
This recipe can be used as a cold main dish during the summer. It can also be garnished with lemon slices and greens and used as an hors d'oeuvre with crackers.

Makes approximately six servings

Approximately 350 calories per serving

■ *Quick Crab Soup*

This is a great family recipe, but I've also often used it for company dinners. If you add a good salad with low-calorie dressing and a sourdough roll, you have an easy, low-calorie supper.

1 can condensed tomato soup (10¾-ounce size)

1 can condensed green pea soup (11¼-ounce size)

2 cans water

1 can crab meat

½ cup sherry

1 dash Worcestershire sauce

Combine soups and water in large saucepan. Add crab meat, sherry, and Worcestershire sauce and heat until it starts to boil. Serve hot.

Serves four

120 calories per serving

■ *The Fish the Coach Caught*

Bud Grant, the former coach of the Minnesota Vikings, is a great fisherman, and his wife is a great cook. The result, this wonderful recipe, was used in *The NFL Cookbook.* The only change I've made is to replace sour cream with yogurt to save calories.

3 pounds walleye pike fillet (or any white fish)

1 cup plain yogurt

¼ cup melted margarine or melted butter

½ teaspoon salt (optional)

½ teaspoon pepper

1 tablespoon chopped parsley

Wipe fillets and pat dry. Place on nonstick, shallow baking pan. Combine next four ingredients and spread over fillets in pan. Bake at 350°F for approximately 30 minutes. Remove from oven and sprinkle with chopped parsley.

Serves five

230 calories per serving

■ Cream of Carrot Soup Without the Cream

You can really make a meal of this! Fill up on it because it is low in calories. (Note: If you must watch your sodium intake, take it easy because canned chicken stock can be very salty. However, there are now some commercial chicken and beef stocks which are low in sodium. Take advantage of them if they're available. Or use your own salt-free stock.)

8 small carrots, chopped or processed fine

1 small chopped onion

2 tablespoons butter

1 bay leaf

3 cups chicken stock

2 teaspoons artificial sweetener

1 tablespoon grated lemon rind

1 tablespoon chopped parsley

Salt and pepper to taste

Combine first three ingredients in heavy saucepan. Cover and cook over low heat until carrots are tender, about 8 to 10 minutes. Add bay leaf and 1 cup of chicken stock. Empty into blender or food processor and blend until liquefied. Return to saucepan and add 2 remaining cups of chicken stock and sweetener. Season with salt and pepper. Pour into soup bowls and garnish with lemon rind and parsley.

Serves six

65 calories per serving

■ Imagine Vichyssoise with Low Calories

We like to serve this great-tasting soup with a good green salad or a baked piece of chicken. This makes a very satisfying winter meal when the soup is served hot, but it's equally delicious—and somewhat more elegant—served cold.

2 tablespoons oil

1 chopped onion

4 cups canned or homemade chicken broth

2 large, peeled and thinly sliced potatoes

2 cups low-fat cottage cheese

1 cup skim milk

1 tablespoon chopped chives (or chopped onions)

Sauté onion in oil until clear. Stir in chicken broth and potatoes, reduce heat, and allow to simmer until potatoes are cooked. Combine milk and cheese in blender until smooth. Place cheese and milk mixture in large mixing bowl and gently stir in potato-broth mixture, 2 cups at a time. Stir until smooth. Heat to serve warm. Refrigerate to serve chilled. Garnish with chopped chives or chopped onions.

Serves eight

107 calories per serving

■ Beef Soup by Muriel Humphrey Brown

I was lucky enough to meet Muriel Humphrey Brown at a March of Dimes gourmet gala. She won first prize with this recipe, and our family has been making it ever since.

1½ pounds stewing beef or chuck

1 soup bone

1 teaspoon salt (optional)

½ teaspoon pepper

2 bay leaves

5 medium sliced carrots

½ cup chopped onions

1 cup chopped celery

1 cup chopped cabbage

1 no. 2 can Italian-style tomatoes

1 tablespoon Worcestershire sauce

1 cup beef broth*

Pinch of oregano

Cover meat and soup bone with cold water in heavy 3-quart kettle. Add salt, pepper, and bay leaves. Bring to a bubbly stage while preparing vegetables. Turn heat to low and add celery, onions, carrots, and cabbage. Simmer until meat is very tender, or at least 2½ hours. Remove bone and bay leaves. Cut meat into bite-sized pieces. Add tomatoes, Worcestershire sauce, beef broth, and oregano. Simmer for ½ hour longer and serve.

Serves six

286 calories per serving

*Again, I recommend that you substitute low-sodium beef broth if available. Worcestershire sauce is very high in sodium, too.

■ *Fast Lane Broccoli*

This is a real winner. It goes well with a variety of main dishes but is especially good with a plain broiled or baked fish.

½ cup Butter Buds liquid*

1 tablespoon dried parsley flakes

2 teaspoons instant minced onion

1½ teaspoons dillweed

½ teaspoon salt (optional)

10-ounce package frozen chopped broccoli, thawed and drained, or 2 cups chopped fresh broccoli

2 tablespoons sliced pimiento, drained

1 cup croutons, plain

*In case you aren't familiar with Butter Buds granules, I recommend them for all weight-watching fast-laners. They're low-calorie, easy to fix, readily available in most supermarkets, and can be used as a powder or made into a liquid.

■ *Fast Lane Broccoli* (continued)

Prepare Butter Buds liquid in a 2-quart saucepan. Add parsley, onion, dill, salt, and broccoli. Cover and cook over medium heat 5 to 6 minutes or until broccoli is tender. Remove from heat and add pimiento and croutons. Toss to coat and serve immediately.

Serves four

91 calories per serving

■ *Molded Egg Salad*

If you're stuck for a main dish lunch that takes minutes to prepare, try this. Your guests (or your family) will eat happily, thinly ever after.

2 envelopes unflavored gelatin

½ cup cold water

1 cup boiling water

12 hard-boiled eggs, riced or sieved

1 cup low-calorie mayonnaise

1½ teaspoons salt (optional)

⅛ teaspoon pepper

1 tablespoon lemon juice

2 tablespoons chopped green pepper

2 tablespoons chopped pimiento

Soak gelatin in cold water for 10 minutes and dissolve mixture in boiling water. Add all other ingredients. Put into a melon-shaped (or ring) mold, sprayed with Pam cooking spray, and chill thoroughly. Serve on a bed of lettuce with low-calorie Russian dressing.

Serves from six to eight

169 calories for each serving

■ *Poppy Seed Noodles*

All of us crave a good pasta dish now and then—especially when we're weight-watching. Here's a recipe for one that's low in calories and very delicious.

1 tablespoon butter

½ cup slivered almonds

2 tablespoons Butter Buds liquid

8 ounces cooked wide noodles

2 teaspoons poppy seeds

Toss almonds with melted butter. Place in a 250°F oven to brown. Mix Butter Buds liquid with cooked noodles. Add poppy seeds and browned almonds. Toss well.

Serves six

152 calories per serving

■ *Gazpacho*

Cold soups are becoming increasingly popular with most of the fast-laners I know. This one's easy to prepare and makes a delicious summer supper.

1 chopped cucumber

1 green pepper, cooked in boiling water for 5 minutes

1 bunch sliced scallions

4 ribs chopped celery

1 chopped garlic clove

2 cans condensed tomato soup

1½ cups ice water

5 tablespoons wine vinegar

5 tablespoons olive oil

Salt and pepper to taste

Combine chopped vegetables. Add olive oil, soup, and rest of ingredients. Cover and chill thoroughly. Place an ice cube in each bowl, add soup, and serve with a few crisp croutons.

Serves eight

125 calories per serving

■ Nuts to Fish

This recipe was first given to me using butter and macadamia nuts. I find this adaptation just as good and quite a bit lower in calories.

½ cup Butter Buds granules

½ cup shredded or grated Parmesan cheese

4 sole fillets (about 1½ pounds total)

½ cup finely chopped pecans

Freshly ground pepper

Parsley or watercress as garnish

Spread half of the Butter Buds granules in the bottom of a shallow baking pan. Sprinkle with half of the Parmesan cheese. Wipe fish dry with a damp cloth and arrange in a single layer over cheese. Pour remaining Butter Buds over fish. Sprinkle with remaining Parmesan cheese and the pecans. Bake 15 minutes or until brown, basting occasionally with the pan drippings. Serve garnished with parsley or watercress and sprinkle with pepper.

Serves four

221 calories per serving

■ Baked Fish Greek Style

This delicious baked fish is low-calorie in spite of the olive oil because there are so few calories in the haddock and the vegetables. I clipped this recipe from *The Minneapolis Star* years ago and have used it many times since.

1 pound haddock fillets

½ teaspoon salt (optional)

1 ripe peeled and diced tomato

¼ sliced green pepper

½ carrot

3 sprigs parsley, cut fine

¼ cup olive oil

¼ cup fresh lemon juice

Arrange fillets in a lightly oiled, shallow baking dish. Season with salt and sprinkle with vegetables. Stir together oil and lemon juice and pour evenly over fish. Bake at 350°F for 20 to 25 minutes, or until fish flakes easily with fork.

Serves four

167 calories per serving

■ Chicken Breasts in Foil

Here's another recipe I found in *The Minneapolis Star* and used for many tailgate parties during our Kicks days.

1 tablespoon butter

1 tablespoon chopped green onions or shallots

4 chicken breasts

4 pieces foil, 12 by 12 inches

8 fresh mushrooms

½ cup dry white wine

A pinch of thyme or tarragon

Salt to taste

Chopped parsley to taste

Sauté onions and chicken in butter for 1 minute in a skillet. Grease each piece of foil lightly with vegetable oil and place a chicken breast in the center. Put two mushrooms on top of each chicken breast. Fold edges of foil upward to create cooking "pans" out of the foil. Add wine to skillet and deglaze (heat gently while scraping browned bits from bottom of pan). Add seasonings. Pour liquid equally into four foil "pans." Seal edges tightly and bake "pans" at 350°F for 1 hour.

Serves four

205 calories per serving

■ Vegetable Dip

Serve this delicious dip with cut-up vegetables such as cauliflower, celery, cucumber, radishes, zucchini, carrots, or mushrooms. Many

■ *Vegetable Dip* (continued)

supermarkets sell vegetables already cut up for dipping, which busy fast-laners appreciate.

1 cup low-fat cottage cheese

1 tablespoon wine vinegar

2 teaspoons grated onion

½ teaspoon garlic salt

½ teaspoon onion salt

1 teaspoon artificial sweetener

¼ teaspoon curry powder

1 teaspoon horseradish

Mix ingredients in a blender and chill until serving time.

The recipe makes approximately 1 cup of dip.

13 calories per 1 T. serving

■ *Pineapple Sorbet*

If you've been hunting for a dessert that's easy to prepare and one that weight-watching guests will appreciate, look no further.

1 large can sliced pineapple packed in its own juice

Champagne (optional)

Drain pineapple slices and reserve ¼ cup of juice. Arrange pineapple slices on a cookie sheet and freeze until firm. Cut up frozen pineapple and place chunks in blender or food processor along with ¼ cup pineapple juice. Blend until fluffy. Using an ice-cream scoop, spoon out sorbet onto cookie sheet and freeze "balls" of sorbet for several hours or overnight. Remove sorbet from freezer 5 minutes before serving time. Put two balls of sorbet in each dessert goblet and serve. If you like and can stand the extra calories, drizzle with champagne at the table.

Serves four

70 calories per serving (without champagne)
85 calories with 2 T. champagne

■ *Santé Potage*

I've mentioned this wonderful, refreshing French soup in the Fast Lane Business Lunch Diet, French style. It's a light, low-calorie pick-me-up that's very popular in France. Here's how you can make it at home:

½ pound sorrel leaves (available at specialty markets)

1 large onion

¼ pound butter

1 quart chicken broth

3 diced potatoes

½ teaspoon dried rosemary

½ pint skim milk

1 teaspoon chopped chervil

Wash and drain sorrel leaves and cut in strips. Mince onion and sauté in butter with sorrel leaves until wilted. Add broth, diced potatoes, and rosemary and simmer 20 minutes or until potatoes are soft. Puree in blender. Return to pan, add milk, and heat gently. Serve garnished with chervil.

Serves eight

150 calories per 1 cup serving

■ *Stracciatella*

Stracciatella is a first-course soup that's served in many Italian restaurants. It's so low in calories that it makes a nice filler-upper before almost any Italian meal.

1 quart chicken broth

2 eggs

2 tablespoons freshly grated Parmesan cheese

2 teaspoons finely chopped parsley

⅛ teaspoon grated nutmeg

Salt to taste

In a small bowl beat eggs slightly and add the cheese, parsley, nutmeg, and salt. In a heavy 2-quart saucepan bring the chicken

■ *Stracciatella* (continued)

broth to a boil. Add the egg mixture, stirring constantly. Simmer and stir for 2 minutes until the egg mixture forms small flakes. Serve garnished with diced spinach if you like.

Serves six

49 calories per 1 cup serving

14

ALTERNATE ROUTES FOR FAST-LANERS WHO CAN'T DRINK MILK

The basic Fast Lane Diet Drink recipe uses milk as its base. Obviously, this isn't for you if you can't drink milk. But that doesn't mean you can't use the Fast Lane Diet to reach your weight-loss destination. Following are two alternate recipes that I think you will like very much, and they're every bit as effective.

■ *No-Milk Diet Drink 1*

 6 ounces (¾ cup) orange juice

 ½ teaspoon corn oil

 ½ banana or another fruit*

 4 crushed ice cubes

 Whirl in blender. Eat with a spoon.

This Diet Drink recipe makes one serving containing approximately 140 calories, depending on the fruit you choose to add. In other words, it's even lower in calories than the basic Diet Drink!

---

*For fruit variations, see recipes in Chapter 4. But the drink tastes best with bananas.

■ *No-Milk Diet Drink 2*

½ cup apple juice (unsweetened)

½ teaspoon corn oil

½ banana or another fruit

4 crushed ice cubes

Whirl in blender. Eat with a spoon.

This Diet Drink recipe also makes one serving and contains approximately 129 calories—again fewer than the basic Diet Drink.

Even if you *can* drink milk, you may want to consider switching to a No-Milk Diet Drink every once in a while. You'll cut your calorie intake almost in half while enjoying the freshness of an all-fruit drink.

Don't hesitate to try your own variations. Almost any unsweetened juice will do nicely for a base. Add zing with half a teaspoon of cinnamon or a fruit extract. Remember that one of the biggest benefits of the Fast Lane Diet Drink is its almost endless number of possible flavors. You don't have to sacrifice taste just because you're forced to take a detour around milk.

If milk is off limits to you, you're not alone. I was surprised to find out how many people have trouble with a substance that many of us take for granted. (I was also surprised to discover how many foods contain milk or milk products—more about that in a minute.)

Over *30 million Americans* today must monitor their milk intake for one of two reasons. Either they're genuinely allergic to milk, or they have a condition known as *lactose intolerance*, which is sometimes mistaken for a milk allergy.

A milk allergy is an abnormal physical reaction to the presence of milk in the body. A lactose intolerance, on the other hand, is the inability to digest milk properly—and it isn't at all abnormal. It is not a disease, even though it may make you feel sick.

If your doctor has diagnosed you as lactose-intolerant, you know what happens when you drink milk or eat a food containing milk. Symptoms range from a mild stomachache all the way to severe diarrhea. Somewhere in between are cramps, gas, a "belchy" feeling, and bloating. You may start reacting to milk within an hour after ingesting it, or it may take several days, depending on your own personal tolerance level.

The reason for lactose intolerance is chemical. Lactose is a disaccharide—double sugar—that must be broken down into two simple sugars, glucose and galactose, before it can be digested. The substance that breaks down the lactose is called lactase, and it's manufactured in the intestines. If your body doesn't make lactase, then milk actually ferments inside your intestines because your body can't handle it.

Luckily, most babies are born with plenty of lactase. But many start losing their ability to digest milk not long after they are weaned. For some, this process levels off, and they never know the difference. For others, it can become a problem down the road.

Certain ethnic groups seem especially likely to develop lactose intolerance. While it's estimated that 20 percent of all white Americans have this condition, the numbers jump to 75 to 90 percent of all black Americans, native Americans, and Asians.

What accounts for the ethnic connection? Nobody knows for sure, but scientists have developed a theory. Lactose intolerance seems to be hereditary. It turns up most often in groups in which, historically, there was not much milk in the diet after infancy. If you're Jewish or of Mediterranean ancestry, you're more likely to be lactose-intolerant than your English or Irish or Scandinavian or German neighbors.

Some people can drink milk all their lives—until they have a bout with a bacterial or viral infection. Or until they take a drug that robs their intestines of lactase. If you develop any of the symptoms described above or any others that concern you, see your doctor.

When you think of milk products, you probably picture the most obvious ones: cheese, yogurt, cream, ice cream, butter. But lactose-intolerant fast-laners have to be alert for potholes: foods in which lactose is "hidden." Following are some things to avoid.

*   *   *

107

- Beverages and mixes made with milk, such as powdered cocoa.

- Bakery goods—including most commercial breads. A welcome exception: kosher breads. Watch out for soda crackers; they may contain lactose as a sweetener.

- Dry or instant cereals, even before you douse them with milk.

- Sherbets (which you shouldn't be eating anyway) are usually made with milk.

- Eggs—if they're scrambled or souffléed with milk.

- Some salad dressings, especially the creamy ones.

- Some fruits, canned or frozen, may contain lactose.

- Some meats, particularly prepared meats, may contain dried milk as a "filler." Hot dogs, for example.

- Soups such as bisques, chowder, or cream soups.

- Sauces and gravies.

- Potatoes mashed with milk or cream.

- Packaged dinners are likely to contain margarine, dried milk, or other milk products.

Tip: Watch out for *anything* creamy, *anything* powdered, *anything* instant, *anything* prepared.

Here's something I never would have guessed: Some vitamin capsules and medications have lactose fillers!

And keep an eye out for additives made from the protein of cow's milk. These include casein, sodium caseinate, and lactalbumin. If you're lactose-intolerant, these may not bother you; if you're allergic to milk, stay away.

How can you find out whether a canned or packaged food product contains the culprit lactose? Usually it's a matter of reading the label. The way in which information is presented on a label is strictly governed by federal regulations. The rule is that whatever there's the most of must be listed first, with the others following in descending order. Fast-laners can usually tell at a glance whether something they don't want to eat is present in significant quantities.

To find out if vitamins or medications contain lactose, you

may have to dig deeper since it may not be mentioned on the label. When in doubt, ask your doctor or pharmacist.

Now for the good news: an abbreviated list of foods you *can* eat if you're lactose-intolerant. Pay attention to calories.

- Almost anything kosher—unless it's marked "kosher dairy."
- Diet Imperial, Mazola Salt-Free, and Weight Watchers margarines; they're all milk-free.
- Some milk substitutes (if you insist), including nondairy whipped toppings.
- Bosco.
- Fish and seafood.
- Bouillons and consommés.
- Pastas.
- Fruit drinks—like the two No-Milk Diet Drinks.
- Grains.
- Fresh vegetables.

If you must cut milk out of your diet, you'll have to make up for the vitamins and minerals you'll lose. Especially important are calcium, the B-complex vitamins, and vitamins C and D.

Calcium is vital for keeping your bones and teeth healthy and strong. Unfortunately, the major source of calcium for most people—except lactose-intolerant fast-laners—is milk. You can get small quantities of it elsewhere in foods like tofu (bean curd), turnip greens, collard greens, rhubarb, salmon, spinach, and broccoli. Your best bet, however, is to take a calcium supplement. Consult your doctor.

The B-complex vitamins—examples are thiamine, riboflavin, and niacin—benefit your brain and nervous system. Any decent over-the-counter multivitamin tablet, taken daily, should satisfy this requirement.

Vitamin C can be found in lots of foods besides milk. The most obvious are citrus fruits and juices—oranges, grapefruit, grapes.

Vitamin D helps your body to use calcium, among the other jobs it does. Small amounts are found in eggs, fish, and meat, but these probably won't be enough to satisfy your daily requirement. Consider taking a supplement but only after you talk with your doctor; too much of this good thing can be toxic.

Fast-laners with lactose intolerance may not have to give up milk and milk products altogether. If you know that you have this condition, all you may need to do is identify those dairy products you can eat without uncomfortable side effects. For example, here are some cheeses that have only traces of lactose: brick, Brie, Camembert, cheddar, cottage cheese (not the creamed kind), Edam, Gouda, provolone, and Stilton.

Can't stand the thought of living without milk? Then there's one more alternative you may want to consider after clearing it with your doctor. (*DO NOT try this if you have a milk allergy!*)

There are products on the market that hydrolyze—or "digest"—lactose for you ahead of time. One is named Lact-Aid. These products come in liquid or powder form, and you can add them to premixed dry skim milk before letting it sit in the refrigerator.

The longer you wait, the more lactose is converted into the two sugars your body can deal with. After twenty-four hours, about 70 percent of the lactose has been hydrolyzed; this rises to about 90 percent after three or four days. You can speed up this process by using more of the product or by heating the milk according to the instructions provided.

Treated milk will taste sweeter than untreated milk, so you may be able to bypass the artificial sweetener when preparing the basic Diet Drink. *Follow the label directions carefully*, including those that tell you how to handle and refrigerate the milk properly afterward.

In some parts of the country, prepared low-lactose milk is available in stores. If you can't find it, check with your pharmacist about the liquid or powder. Then try this variation.

■ *Basic Diet Drink with Low-Lactose Milk*

2 cups treated milk

2 teaspoons corn oil

1 teaspoon vanilla extract

1 packet artificial sweetener (optional)

This recipe makes two servings of the Fast Lane Diet Drink for people with a moderate lactose intolerance. *Stop drinking it immediately if you experience any discomfort at all.*

Some of my friends have asked me why I don't recommend the use of soy "milk." Personally, I hate the taste. But go ahead and experiment with it if you like.

■ *Basic Diet Drink with Soy Bean Milk*

2 cups soy bean milk

2 teaspoons corn oil

1 teaspoon vanilla extract

1 teaspoon imitation sweetener

Combine and mix thoroughly; if you like, whirl in blender or mix in shaker till foamy.

This recipe makes about 2 cups of basic Diet Drink. Each cup contains 74 calories.

When all is said and done, I stick to my original recommendations: the two No-Milk Diet Drinks. They're easy, they're quick, they work—and that's what the Fast Lane Diet is all about.

15

THE FAST LANE VITAMIN CHECKLIST

Those of us who live in the fast lane use more of certain vitamins and minerals faster than people with calmer, less demanding lives. That's part of the price we pay for success. Fortunately, supplements are readily available, and doctors and scientists are constantly adding to their store of knowledge about these essential nutrients. So it's not hard to get what we need to keep our engines running.

The Fast Lane Diet gives you more than a way to lose weight quickly and easily; it's nutritionally sound.

Here's what's in it for you:

Each serving of the basic Diet Drink supplies 20 grams of protein.

The U.S. recommended daily allowance (RDA) of protein for a 120-pound woman is 43 grams; for a 170-pound man, it's 61 grams.

Each serving of the basic Diet Drink supplies 38.4 grams of carbohydrates.

Although there's no official U.S. RDA for carbohydrates, it's believed that a minimum of 50 grams per day is needed.

Carbohydrates have gotten a lot of bad press lately, and they don't deserve it. The truth is that carbohydrates supply most of our energy. They only cause problems when we consume too many of them—when they turn into fat. Gram for gram, they have the same number of calories as protein!

Each serving of the basic Diet Drink supplies 9 grams of fat.

For a variety of reasons, we all need some fat in our diets. Fat deposits in muscles are a source of energy. They're especially important for the heart muscle. Fat in our bodies protects our delicate inner organs. The oils in fats keep our complexions glowing and our hair silky. And fats help build prostaglandins, essential both to cell membranes and for regulating the body's use of cholesterol.

Most Americans consume six to eight times as much fat as they need. A lot of it is the wrong kind—saturated animal fats, which raise the cholesterol level in the blood.

In developing the Fast Lane Diet Drink, I paid close attention to the fat content. That's why I used only skim milk and corn oil. In skim milk, almost all the fat has been removed. Corn oil is a liquid vegetable oil containing polyunsaturated fats, the kind doctors recommend because they seem to keep the lid on blood pressure.

What about vitamins and minerals? The basic Diet Drink offers plenty of what you need in those areas, too. Here's a breakdown of the percentages of the U.S. RDAs in each serving:

	Percent RDA
Protein	50
Vitamin A	25
Vitamin C	5
Thiamine (vitamin B-1)	15
Riboflavin (vitamin B-2)	62.5
Pantothenic acid (vitamin B-5)	20

	Percent RDA
Vitamin B-6	10
Vitamin B-12	50
Vitamin D	62.5
Calcium	75.5
Phosphorus	62.5
Magnesium	15

NOTE: These figures refer *only* to the basic Diet Drink. When you vary the recipe by adding fruits, eggs, and extracts, you increase the nutritional content.

Now let's look at a few of the things each vitamin does for your body.

Vitamin A: Ever wonder about the connection between carrots and good eyesight? Well, it's not just an old wives' tale—it's fact. This is because carrots are rich in vitamin A, which is necessary for vision in dim light. Vitamin A is also essential to healthy skin, hair, and mucous membranes. It promotes normal bone growth and development and normal reproduction and builds resistance to respiratory infections. And it's possible that it helps prevent cancers of the skin, lungs, and bladder.

Vitamin C: Probably the vitamin you've heard the most about—whether it prevents or alleviates cold symptoms is still up for grabs—vitamin C plays a big part in the formation of collagen. Collagen is important for the growth and repair of tissue cells, capillaries, teeth, and bones. Vitamin C also protects other vitamins from oxidation, the process that breaks them down before your body has the chance to get the most out of them. And it helps your body absorb iron.

Thiamine (vitamin B-1): Known as the "morale vitamin," thiamine keeps your nervous system in shape and can improve your mental attitude. It also helps release the energy locked into the carbohydrates you eat.

Riboflavin (vitamin B-2): Riboflavin does most of its work at the cell level, promoting normal growth and reproduction. It keeps your skin, eyes, nails, and hair healthy. Riboflavin de-

THE FAST LANE DIET

ficiency is the most common vitamin deficiency among Americans today. Its signs are scaly or cracked skin, especially around the mouth, and sensitivity to light.

Pantothenic Acid: Important to cell building, normal growth, and the central nervous system. It helps your body to metabolize carbohydrates, proteins, and fats.

Vitamin B-6: Vitamin B-6 helps your body absorb and use proteins and fats. It aids in the production of red blood cells and some hormones and is important to healthy teeth and gums.

Vitamin B-12: The "red vitamin" is important to the formation of red blood cells and genetic material. It also helps your nervous and digestive systems function properly.

Vitamin D: Your body makes vitamin D—the "sunshine vitamin"—all by itself when sun shines on your skin. This vitamin helps in the absorption of calcium and phosphorus for strong bones and teeth.

Calcium: Ninety-nine percent of the calcium in your body is found in your bones and teeth. This is the mineral that helps prevent osteoporosis—the thinning of the bones that often comes with age. Calcium works with magnesium to promote cardiovascular health and keep your heart beating regularly. It's also involved in blood clotting, enzyme and hormone activities, and sound sleep.

Phosphorus: Like calcium, the mineral phosphorus is concentrated in your bones and teeth. It also plays a major part in the functioning of your cells, and it helps to metabolize energy-giving fats and starches.

Magnesium: The "antistress mineral," magnesium fights depression, helps prevent heart attacks, and helps prevent kidney stones and gallstones.

There are other vitamins and minerals not contained in the basic Diet Drink that you should be sure to get enough of. Any one of the six Fast Lane Diet plans should satisfy your body's daily requirements for vitamins E, K, B-3 (niacin), H (biotin), and folic acid. And it should take care of your greater-than-usual needs for iron, sulfur, sodium, chlorine, and so on.

Still, we fast-laners owe it to ourselves to make absolutely sure that we're getting everything our overworked bodies need to stay healthy. That's why I take a high-potency time-release multiple vitamin plus a mineral tablet plus a vitamin C supplement—every day. So should you, no matter which of the diet plans you follow. And even when you've reached your goal, keep taking them!

When I first started getting serious about getting in shape for my fast lane life, I had a lot of questions about vitamins. I'll share what I found out with you.

1. Is there any difference between natural and synthetic vitamins?

Surprisingly—no. The chemical formulas are the same, and your body uses both kinds in exactly the same way. So don't bother wasting time (something fast-laners have too little of as it is) chasing around to health food stores. Buy your vitamins at your local pharmacy—or stock up at a discount store.

Natural vitamins cost more, but they don't do more. That's good news for your wallet.

2. Can vitamins be too much of a good thing?

Only if you overdo it on certain ones. Megadoses can be poisonous to your system.

Basically, there are two "types" of vitamins—the *water-solubles* and the *fat-solubles.*

The water-solubles—all eight B-complex vitamins plus C—are constantly being used up or washed out of your body. You need to replenish your supply of each on a daily basis. If you take too much of any one, your body will usually get rid of the excess on its own.

The fat-solubles—A, D, E, and K—are stored in body fat. It's not absolutely necessary to consume them daily unless you're getting only marginal amounts in your diet. But because they're stored, not excreted or sweated out, they can build up to toxic levels if you overdo them. Fast-laners have a tendency to overdo almost everything, so watch out.

It's strange, but a lot of people who are otherwise very

117

careful about what they eat and drink seem to lose their good judgment when it comes to vitamins. They avoid processed foods because they don't want to be "contaminated" by chemicals, and then they turn around and gobble vitamins. *Vitamins are chemicals, too,* even "natural" ones.

Not to scare you, but to make this absolutely clear, here's a rundown of the toxic side effects of a few of the more popular vitamins:

- Too much vitamin A over several months can lead to hair loss, nausea, blurred vision, scaly skin, fatigue, splitting headaches, and an enlarged liver—to name just a few of the nastier symptoms.

- Too much vitamin D can cause deafness, kidney stones, high blood pressure, vomiting, diarrhea, sore eyes, and itchy skin. It can also result in calcium deposits in the liver, lungs, kidney, stomach, and blood-vessel walls—which may be mistaken for cancer.

- You thought that gout went out with the Victorian novel. Wrong! It may be a side effect of too much niacin (vitamin B-3).

In addition, vitamins, like medications, can act on one another in unpleasant ways. Not even the water-solubles are innocent when it comes to this sort of thing. For example, an excess of any B-complex vitamin can deplete the others. And megadoses of vitamin C can flush B-12 and folic acid out of your body before they have the chance to work.

Never take a megadose of anything before consulting your doctor. And try to ascertain that your doctor is knowledgeable about vitamins and their effects—both the risks and the benefits.

3. Does it matter at what time of the day I take my vitamins?

You don't want to down your vitamins just before you go to bed for the night. You'll lose the benefits of having them course through your bloodstream while you're active.

If you have a lot on your mind during the day—fast-laners usually do—then you might want to take them in the morning, when you're standing in front of the bathroom mirror. That way you're more likely to make them a habit.

However, you should know that the *best* time to take vitamins, if you simply must take them all at once, is after the largest meal of the day—probably dinner. A vitamin consumed immediately following a meal is absorbed better than one dropped into an empty stomach. Think of it as dessert!

If at all possible, though, you should spread the dosage out over intervals throughout the day.

4. Is it necessary to take the exact U.S. RDA for each nutrient?

The "R" in RDA means "recommended," not "required." U.S. RDAs are only *estimates* of what *healthy* people need. Your needs will depend on your height, weight, occupation, physical condition, mental condition, activity level, stress level, and so on.

Fast-laners do everything at top speed. I tend to believe— and the health professionals I've consulted agree—that the RDAs aren't sufficient for fast-laners. Because you do more, you deserve more. Pay attention to what your body tells you—and get your doctor's advice before going too far overboard.

5. I have trouble swallowing pills. Are vitamins available in other forms?

Of course. You can purchase powders and liquids and mix them right in with your Fast Lane Diet Drink.

Powders tend to be more potent than tablets or capsules. And they usually don't come with fillers, binders, or additives, so they're better for people with allergies (or people who simply want to avoid fillers, binders, or additives).

If you can take pills comfortably, though, I'd recommend tablets or capsules simply because they're easier to deal with. They also hold their potency longer than powders or liquids.

6. Do vitamins ever go "bad"?

If you store your vitamins in a cool, dark place out of direct sunlight and keep the lids on tight, most of them and your

mineral supplements will last up to a year after being opened—
or two to three years if they're left sealed. So go ahead and take
advantage of that annual sale.

Most packaged vitamins come with expiration dates stamped
on their labels. Very old vitamins probably won't poison you,
but they won't do you much good either. Toss them and treat
yourself to a brand-new bottle.

7. Is it OK to skip a meal and take vitamins instead?

No—for a number of reasons.

First, vitamins aren't "pep" pills. They can't give you energy
all by themselves; they work in combination with proteins, carbohydrates, and fats.

Second, as I said earlier, vitamins are absorbed better if
they're taken after meals. Otherwise, they go in one end and
out the other.

And third, skipping meals is a bad idea at any time, especially when you're dieting. You're more susceptible to the munchies—and more likely to eat irresponsibly just to satisfy the
gnawing monster in your stomach.

* * *

If we lived in a squeaky-clean world, and if we ate perfectly
balanced diets, and if we didn't have any bad habits, then we
wouldn't need vitamin and mineral supplements. But we don't,
and we don't, and we do, so we do.

Fast-laners who pay attention to what they eat and drink
can control their intake of less-than-desirable substances. But
unless you want to walk around wearing a gas mask, there's
nothing you can do about the air you breathe.

Each year, literally hundreds of tons of pollutants—many
potentially harmful—are belched or leaked or exuded into the
atmosphere by factory stacks, automobile exhaust pipes, incin-
erators, power plants, chemical dumps, refineries, and the like.
You breathe them in through your nose and mouth. You absorb
them through your skin.

Your job may be hazardous to your health—if you're a printer,
or an electrical engineer, or a paperhanger, or a mechanic, or
a dental hygienist, and on and on. Even if you're a secretary in

a no-smoking office, you may be breathing dangerous fumes from duplicating machines or ozone from a switchboard.

The *antioxidants*—vitamins A, C, E, and selenium—afford about the best protection you can get against these invisible enemies. Vitamin A protects your mucous membranes; vitamin C battles bacterial infections; vitamin E functions as an anti-pollutant in the lungs. And research has shown that the presence of selenium in the blood may have something to do with cancer prevention. In addition, all these vitamins help each other out.

If you haven't taken your vitamins today, go do it *this instant*.

Now let's talk about bad habits—and not-bad habits—that may jeopardize your health and cancel the vitamins you take.

Cigarettes

Too many fast-laners are smokers. I'm not going to tell you to quit because whether or not you smoke is your business, but I am going to tell you how to counteract at least one of the harmful effects.

The Canadian government performed a two-year study of smokers that resulted in some very important findings. In brief: *People who smoke a pack and a half of cigarettes a day have 30 to 40 percent less vitamin C in their blood than nonsmokers.*

Here's another interesting statistic: Each cigarette destroys 25 milligrams of vitamin C.

Ever wonder why smokers tend to get colds more often than nonsmokers? Nobody has yet proved beyond any doubt that vitamin C either cures or prevents colds—but it's certainly a coincidence worth noticing.

If you smoke, you need twice the RDA of vitamin C than the average adult who doesn't smoke. That's a fact.

Alcohol

A glass of wine with dinner or a Scotch-on-the-rocks before or a martini at lunch—each of these is part of many fast-laners' lifestyles. Try not to drink while on any of the Fast Lane Diet plans.

You know that alcohol is nothing but empty calories. But

as long as you imbibe in extreme moderation, you shouldn't have to worry about weight gain. See the official Fast Lane Diet Cocktail recipe earlier in the book on page 54.

If you go overboard frequently, however, you're going to need more thiamine (vitamin B-1), niacin (vitamin B-3), vitamin B-6, and folic acid than your teetotaler friends. Excessive alcohol consumption will do a number on your liver and interfere with its ability to store and use vitamins. It will also prevent your body from absorbing the vitamins you would otherwise get from the foods you eat.

Finally, some vitamins that would otherwise go to process food will be sidetracked into processing the alcohol—or repairing damaged tissue.

If you consume four or more shots of alcohol each day, you will definitely need a multivitamin supplement. And you may need additional individual supplements if you're not eating properly—another common problem with drinkers.

Caffeine

Coffee, tea, cola drinks, and chocolate beverages can rob your system of some of the B-complex vitamins it needs. And besides, caffeine is a drug. Fast-laners may think they need the high it provides; but they certainly don't need the let-down that follows.

Television

While it hasn't been proved that too much TV will deprive you of anything but your native intelligence, it can put a strain on your eyes and create the need for some extra vitamins A and D.

Birth-control Pills

Oral contraceptives can lead to shortages of several water-soluble vitamins, among them B-1, B-2, B-6, B-12, C, and folic acid.

Other Drugs and Medications

Over-the-counter and prescription drugs alike can influence how vitamins behave in your body—and how much of them are left to work on your behalf.

If you take a lot of aspirin, your digestive tract lining may be damaged to the point where it cannot absorb certain nutrients.

If you're on antibiotics for a long period of time, the intestinal bacteria that produce vitamin K and some of the B-complex vitamins may be destroyed.

Megadoses of vitamins can also impede the action of certain drugs you're taking for a medical problem. Ask your doctor.

The Fast Lane Diet—or Any Other

If you're cutting back on your calorie intake, you *must* balance the scale on the other side by taking supplements. Otherwise, you may end up lethargic or ill.

Jet Lag: A Particular Problem for Fast-Laners

There are ways to alleviate the fatigue, disorientation, and general sense of crumminess that go hand in hand with heavy air travel.

Drink lots of liquids—but avoid caffeine so you can catnap if you need to.

Take one gram of vitamin C for each time zone you cross. Add thiamine (vitamin B-1) to keep your mind alert. Finally, supplement the traveler's traditional low-fiber diet with bran.

Fast-laners are special people with special nutritional needs. They tend to abuse their bodies and ignore them when they cry for help. Fast-laners eat too many carbohydrates and starches. They experience ups and downs in dizzying succession. They suffer from stress and anxiety.

For some fast-laners, the supplements I recommend—one high-potency time-release multiple vitamin plus a mineral tablet plus a vitamin C supplement—won't be sufficient to keep them humming along in perfect tune. They're going to need more of some things, less of others.

Here are some suggestions for people in specific circumstances. Again, talk to your doctor before deciding on what and how much to take.

Women over the age of 25 have special calcium and iron needs. The Fast Lane Diet Drink is rich in calcium, so if you use the drink two or three times a day, you should be fine in that area. But if you feel tired, consider taking extra iron. (Iron toxicity is extremely rare in adults.)

People under pressure or those in especially demanding positions should counteract the effects of stress with stress–B-complex vitamins sold over the counter (for example, Stress-tabs). Vitamin B-15 (pangamic acid) has been studied extensively in the Soviet Union, and the claim is made that it can lengthen the lives of cells, quell the craving for liquor (an occupational hazard for some executive types), and alleviate hangovers.

People on weird or irregular schedules—students, air traffic controllers, police officers, or anyone who must sometimes sacrifice sleep to a swing shift or a deadline—can take the edge off with stress–B-complex vitamins and extra vitamin E. Try not to skip meals entirely. Pack your Fast Lane Diet Drink in a thermos and take it with you. If you work the night shift often, add vitamin D and tryptophan (an essential amino acid).

People whose jobs—or avocations—are physically demanding need more carbohydrates and protein than the rest of us whose lives are less frenetic. Stress–B-complex vitamins, extra vitamins C and E, more minerals, and occasional protein supplements are recommended. Calcium and magnesium (for your overworked bones) are also worth considering.

People whose jobs expose them to hazardous substances (and that could be anybody these days) should beef up their diets with vitamins A, C, and E (they help "detoxify" your body) and supplement them with a B-complex boost.

People who come into frequent contact with the public will benefit from a stress–B-complex plus vitamin E. If you're in sales, this should help put punch in your presentation. If you're in medicine, you need extra protection: Try a double dose of the stress–B-complex, plus vitamin C. And if you're a teacher, you'll need the added energy the stress–B-complex provides.

The best way to develop your own vitamin regimen involves two steps: Educate yourself on the virtues of the various nutrients and pay attention to what your body is telling you. Then put two and two together, in consultation with your doctor, to come up with the plan that's right for you.

16

COUNTING THE CALORIES YOU BURN WHILE LIVING AND WORKING IN THE FAST LANE

Americans are getting fatter every year—despite the new focus on thinness and fitness. The average American man weighs 20 to 30 pounds more than he should; the average American woman packs 15 to 30 pounds more than she should on her smaller frame. Even children are overweight.

What's your ideal weight? The charts that follow, prepared by insurance companies, will give you some approximate figures. In all cases, the weights shown are based on mortality rates; in other words, they are associated with the longest life expectancies.

Charts 1 and 2, from the Metropolitan Life Insurance Company, can help you determine your ideal weight according to your height and the size of your frame.

* * *

1. Weight in Pounds by Height and Frame Size for Men, Ages 25–59

Height	Small frame	Medium frame	Large frame
5'2"	128–134	131–141	138–150
5'3"	130–136	133–143	140–153
5'4"	132–138	135–145	142–156
5'5"	134–140	137–148	144–160
5'6"	136–142	139–151	146–164
5'7"	138–145	142–154	149–168
5'8"	140–148	145–157	152–172
5'9"	142–151	148–160	155–176
5'10"	144–154	151–163	158–180
5'11"	146–157	154–166	161–184
6'0"	149–160	157–170	164–188
6'1"	152–164	160–174	168–192
6'2"	155–168	164–178	172–197
6'3"	158–172	167–182	176–202
6'4"	162–176	171–187	181–207

NOTE: The above heights assume shoes with 1-inch heels; the weights include 5 pounds of clothing.

2. Weight in Pounds by Height and Frame Size for Women, Ages 25–59

Height	Small frame	Medium frame	Large frame
4'10"	102–111	109–121	118–131
4'11"	103–113	111–123	120–134
5'0"	104–115	113–126	122–137
5'1"	106–118	115–129	125–140
5'2"	108–121	118–132	128–143
5'3"	111–124	121–135	131–147
5'4"	114–127	124–138	134–151
5'5"	117–130	127–141	137–155
5'6"	120–133	130–144	140–159
5'7"	123–136	133–147	143–163
5'8"	126–139	136–150	146–167
5'9"	129–142	139–153	149–170

Height	Small frame	Medium frame	Large frame
5'10"	132–145	142–156	153–173
5'11"	135–148	145–159	155–176
6'0"	138–151	148–162	158–179

NOTE: The above heights assume shoes with 1-inch heels; the weights include 3 pounds of clothing.

Charts 3 and 4, from the Pacific Mutual Life Insurance Company, break ideal weights into age categories. Although the starting weights are somewhat lower than those recommended by Metropolitan, I prefer this way of presenting information because it seems more realistic to me. Most people, even those in perfect shape, tend to gain some weight as they get older. But not much, as you'll see.

3. Average Weight in Pounds by Height and Age for Men, Ages 20–69

Height	Age 20–29	Age 30–39	Age 40–49	Age 50–59	Age 60–69
5'3"	125	129	130	131	130
5'6"	135	140	142	143	142
5'9"	149	153	155	156	155
6'0"	161	166	167	168	167
6'3"	176	181	183	184	180

4. Average Weight in Pounds by Height and Age for Women, Ages 20–69

Height	Age 20–29	Age 30–39	Age 40–49	Age 50–59	Age 60–69
4'10"	97	102	106	109	111
5'1"	106	109	114	118	120
5'4"	114	118	122	127	129
5'7"	123	127	132	137	140
5'10"	134	138	142	146	147

Whatever your personal ideal weight may be—and this is something you should determine in consultation with your doctor—the Fast Lane Diet can help you to reach it easily and quickly. How quickly is up to you. Specifically, it's a function of how active you are; I'll talk more about that in a moment.

But first, you should understand that successful dieting is always a matter of checks and balances. If you consume more calories than you use, you gain weight. If your consumption and use are equal, your weight stays the same. It's only when your output exceeds your input that you start seeing real results. At that point, your body begins drawing on its own fat reserves—the energy stored up in fat deposits on your waist, your stomach, your back end, your thighs, your upper arms, wherever.

You've reached your ideal weight when your body consists of 5 to 10 percent fat if you're a man or 10 to 20 percent fat if you're a woman. Of course, you won't be able to measure that yourself—you won't be able to look inside your body and determine the percentages. But you will be able to look into a mirror, and your mirror won't lie.

To take off a single pound of fat, you must burn roughly 3,500 calories *more* than you take in over a given period of time. The average person burns between 1,500 and 2,700 calories per day on normal activities. Weight loss occurs when those 1,500 to 2,700 calories amount to more than the total number of calories you're ingesting.

If you haven't been able to lose weight until now, the reason is very simple: You've struck the balance between your calorie input and output that maintains your weight where it is. What you want to do now is tip that balance in your favor. And the way to accomplish that is by cutting down on the calories you consume and by stepping up the calories you use.

I want to say a few words here about going overboard. Fast-laners have that tendency. When they want something, they want it *now*. They don't let anything stand in their way.

This can cause problems on both the input and output sides of the diet equation. On the input side, some fast-laners start dieting by going "cold turkey" on food: They fast. There are several reasons why I do not recommend fasting.

Even if you eat nothing for two whole days, it would take nearly that long to lose just one pound of bona fide body fat.

You might appear to lose more—your scale might tell you something different—but in truth you'd be losing water weight, not fat weight. As soon as you started eating again, you'd gain it back.

It's difficult and uncomfortable to go without eating for days at a stretch.

You get hungry and cranky and weak. Your concentration begins to falter—all you can think about is food! You slow down—something people who live in the fast lane can't afford to do.

And, most important, you jeopardize your health.

Doctors have linked fasting to depression and, in some cases, death. *Don't risk it for benefits that are temporary and hazards whose effects may be long-lasting or permanent.*

The Fast Lane Fast is not a true fast because it provides you with all the nutritional advantages of the Fast Lane Diet Drink four times a day.

Fast-laners have been known to jump into exercise programs without really knowing what they're doing. This can result in consequences ranging from mild stiffness and discomfort to serious injuries. *If you are not accustomed to strenuous exercise, you should not begin it without first having a complete physical and discussing your planned program with your doctor.*

Any of the Fast Lane Diet plans will help you from the start by cutting your daily calorie intake in half or more, depending on which plan you follow and on how much you're accustomed to eating when you're not dieting. (For example, Fast Lane Diet

Plan 1 will reduce your calorie intake to 840 to 950 calories per day.)

From the very first day, in other words, your body will be forced to draw on its fat reserves for the energy it needs even if you're not particularly active. That's because your body burns calories even when it's totally at rest. It takes energy to perform the vital functions of keeping your heart pumping, your lungs expanding and contracting, your digestive system working, your kidneys filtering blood, your cells making essential chemicals, and so on.

All the charts show the approximate calorie costs of the activities listed when each is done for one hour. Estimates are for weights ranging from 150 to 175 pounds.

When compiling your own daily "totals," keep in mind that each pound of excess body fat is the equivalent of 3,500 calories of energy that needs to be spent!

5. Calories Burned per Hour on Sedentary or Light Activities

Activity	Calories
Sleeping	67
Thinking	80
Sitting	84
Studying	90
Standing (relaxed)	93
Sitting in class	100
Eating, reading	100
Playing the piano	135
Driving a car	147
Getting dressed	225

6. Calories Burned per Hour on Work-Related Activities

Activity	Calories
Writing	99
Typing	103
Bartending	183

Activity	Calories
Painting	218
Radio/TV repair	222
Carpentry (light)	228
Assembly line work, stocking shelves	257
Waitress duties	270
Driving a truck	294
Busboy duties	335
Manual labor	420
Heavy labor	810

7. Calories Burned per Hour on Housework

Activity	Calories
Sewing	99
Ironing, washing dishes	132
Cooking dinner	150
Dusting, sweeping the floor	172
Cleaning windows, mopping floors, vacuuming	270
Scrubbing floors	330
Climbing stairs	609

8. Calories Burned per Hour on Other Around-the-House Activities

Activity	Calories
Working on the car, washing the car	183
Riding a lawn mower	195
Pushing a light power mower	270
Gardening	367
Pushing a hand mower	450
Sawing wood	540
Shoveling heavy snow	1,170

9. Calories Burned per Hour on Light Recreational Activities

Activity	Calories
Playing cards	100
Power boating, shuffleboard	183
Bowling, billiards, fishing, golf (with cart)	222
Horseback riding, archery, sailing	257

10. Calories Burned per Hour on Moderate Recreational Activities

Activity	Calories
Table tennis	294
Bicycling, 5.5 mph	300
Rowing (moderate pace)	312
Calisthenics	315
Tennis (doubles), ballet exercises, badminton, volleyball	330
Golf (no cart)	345
Ballroom dancing	367
Roller skating	390
Badminton	417
Hiking, hunting, square dancing, waterskiing	441
Tennis (singles)	450
Bicycling, 10 mph	519
Swimming, continuous freestyle (slow)	540
Downhill skiing	588

11. Calories Burned per Hour on More Strenuous Recreational Activities

Activity	Calories
Touch football	665
Mountain climbing	690
Squash, handball, racquetball	700

Activity	Calories
Jogging, 5.5 mph	750
Bicycling, 13 mph	760
Trampolining	875
Running, 8 mph	1,008
Cross-country skiing, 10 mph	1,100

Walking has only recently begun to get the credit it deserves as a superb form of exercise. It's easy to do, it doesn't require special equipment or skills, and it usually won't result in injuries common to other more bone-jarring exercises. Swing your arms and pick up your feet and you'll burn up calories at a very respectable rate: around 280 per hour if you walk a moderate 3 mph, 370 or more if you clip along at 4 mph.

The most efficient way to lose weight is by combining a nutritious diet with frequent and regular exercise. There's no way around that simple (if sometimes painful) truth.

It's *possible* to shed pounds while lying flat on your back and taking in the minimum number of calories needed to sustain life, but what will you look like when you've reached your ideal weight? Flabby! Saggy! Wrinkled! Not in the least like that gorgeous actor or actress whose picture you've taped to your refrigerator door.

Sorry, but to look your best you're going to have to work at it. Exercise has other benefits in addition to a sleeker body and improved muscle tone: Your skin will glow. In all probability, you'll prolong your life. And you'll feel better almost immediately: vibrant, energetic, and ready to burn up the miles in the fast lane faster than ever before.

Here are a few tips that should help you to form the exercise habit:

- Instead of taking the elevator, walk up one floor and down two.
- Tell everybody you know about your plans to start exercising. Maybe someone will join you on your daily walk, jog, or swim.
- Join a health club or gym or your local YMCA or YWCA. Once you've paid a membership fee, you'll hate to let the money go to waste.

- Draw up a "fitness contract" for yourself, detailing your exercise program for the coming month, and sign it. In ink!

- Walk whenever possible—to the grocery store, the post office, a friend's house. When shopping, park a few blocks away from your destination.

- If the company you work for offers a fitness program, take advantage of it.

- Make your next vacation an active one. Rather than lying on the beach, hike some hills. Or take up a new sport—cross-country skiing? Horseback riding? Wind surfing?

- Invest in a good pair of walking or running shoes.

- Do floor exercises in front of the evening news.

- Clean your house to the latest dance music. That should get you moving!

- For every half pound you lose, pay yourself a dollar. When you've reached your target weight, splurge on a (nonfood) treat for yourself.

- Take a before-the-new-you picture of yourself and tape it to the inside of your refrigerator. When you're in shape, take a new-you picture, have copies made, and send them to your relatives.

- Come up with your *own* get-in-the-habit tips. Write them down. Then follow your own advice!

17

RULES OF THE ROAD FOR FAST LANE DIETERS: Dos and Don'ts Plus a List of No-Calorie and Low-Calorie Snacks

I used to think that when Robert Louis Stevenson wrote, "The world is so full of a number of things/You'd think that we'd all be as happy as kings," he was talking about food. "A loaf of bread, a jug of wine, and thou" seemed to me the bare bones of a picnic in the making. What it needed was a few embellishments—pâté de foie gras, sweet butter, cheesecake, a decent dry Manhattan.

We fast-laners are surrounded by culinary temptations on all sides. In almost every city I can think of, new restaurants are springing up at an astonishing rate. There are more kinds of things to eat—and more places to eat them in—than ever before. Fast foods are getting tastier and fancier. And with grazing—stopping here for one item, there for another—becoming the convenient, modern way to dine, it's downright difficult to maintain a stiff upper lip, not to mention keeping it clamped over your lower one.

You *want* to lose weight; that's why you've made a commitment to the Fast Lane Diet. But even a road paved with good intentions has its potholes.

That bakery on your way to work with flaky croissants in the window . . . the Häagen Dazs chocolate-chocolate chip you bought "for the kids" . . . the cookie samples that come in the mail . . . the invitation to dinner from a friend who makes Julia Child look like a rookie . . . the late-night urge to finish off the Sara Lee . . . You know what I mean. Sometimes it's easier to succumb and hide your bathroom scale in a closet for a few weeks.

Unlike other diets, the Fast Lane Diet won't wreak havoc with your body chemistry, so it's no big deal if you stray off the straight and narrow once in a while. But the more closely you stick to it, the more quickly it will work for you. And no diet can be effective if it's supplemented with high-calorie snacks.

I'm going to share with you a few tricks that help me take my mind off food. Then I'm going to point you in the direction of some low-calorie munchies for those times when you can't say no.

I've designed the Fast Lane Diet Drink to allow for countless variations and flavors. For the most part, a different Diet Drink should be sufficient to satisfy your craving for different taste sensations. Save time by making the basic Diet Drink in batches and freezing individual portions—then, when it's time for a meal, defrost and add whatever fresh, natural, low-calorie ingredients you have handy.

Follow a blueberry breakfast with a carob lunch. Next day, try banana before an Olympic dinner. The less often you repeat a particular drink (unless you fall madly in love with it), the longer it will take to get bored.

It's my opinion that most diets fail because dieters simply can't stand the thought of them after a while. The Fast Lane Diet has been successful for so many people because it's not the same old thing, day in and day out.

Dos and Don'ts: Tips for Staying on Track

DO notice when you've had enough.

DON'T eat until you're stuffed.

138

DO weigh yourself at least once every twenty-four hours. If you cut your daily intake by about 1,000 calories, you'll lose approximately 2 pounds a week!

DON'T talk on the telephone in or near your kitchen. Since fast-laners tend to do at least two things at once, make sure one of them isn't munching while you're on the phone!

DO move around as much as you can during the day.

DON'T always rely on your secretary, assistant, housekeeper, spouse, or kids to do the physical work around your office or home. Additional physical activity translates into additional calories burned.

DO remember that laughing out loud and hard consumes about 3 calories per minute.

DON'T be a pain just because you're dieting and others around you aren't. Be patient and pleasant and get ready to reap compliments on your new look.

DO take a few deep breaths whenever the thought of food crosses your mind; it will help to curb your appetite.

DON'T expect instant gratification. Most people lose weight gradually, sometimes slowly.

DO remember that *you*, like all fast-laners, *are in control.*

DON'T be hard on yourself if sometimes you lose control. It's only temporary!

DO clear the decks of all fattening foods. Clean out the fridge and cabinets; give away or store the stuff you love but shouldn't indulge in.

DON'T buy more than you need when shopping for the Fast Lane Diet. Picking up large quantities of what's called for may lead to eating them sooner. Fresh fruits and vegetables also lose many of their nutrients when stored.

DO make the necessary rearrangements to your lifestyle to remove temptation. If you're used to snacking in front of the evening news, do stretching exercises instead.

DON'T torture yourself with visions of meals you're missing.

DO take plenty of time to chew and swallow each bite.

DON'T wolf your food. The slower you eat, the faster you fill.

DO go on to something else as soon as you're done eating. Get up from the table and out of the dining room or kitchen.

DON'T ask for seconds of *anything* unless it's water!

DO diet with a partner if at all possible. There's strength in numbers.

DON'T get discouraged if you're a woman and your dieting partner is a man and he loses weight faster than you do. That's normal. First, women need fewer calories. Second, women, as the childbearers of the species, have a permanent subcutaneous layer of fat already built in. And third, women seem to metabolize carbohydrates less efficiently than men. The carbohydrates are converted to fat rather than consumed for energy.

DO change the topic if food comes up in a conversation.

DON'T feel sorry for yourself because you're "doing without" certain things. Think instead of what you'll be able to do with the new you.

DO get your mind off of food by broadening your range of interests.

DON'T take a cooking class!

DO drink *lots* of water, herb teas, and other permitted liquids.

DON'T stoke up on caffeine. It will make you nervous and jittery in addition to negating the positive effects of some vitamins.

DO plan to do something nice for yourself once you reach your goal. (Save the money you'd normally spend on doughnuts or snacks and blow it then.)

DON'T buy yourself a new item of clothing now, in a smaller size, for that day when you achieve your target weight. (Your taste in clothes may change completely once you're walking around in a renovated body. And who knows—you might need an even smaller size!)

DO exercise as often as you can.

DON'T overdo it at the start. Any exercise program should begin gradually and work its way up from there.

DO allow for some spontaneity in your life. Take in a movie at the spur of the moment. Go dancing. Go walking. Visit a friend. Check out the new show at your local art museum.

DON'T limit your social engagements to eating and drinking events.

DO hang pictures of gorgeous models on your refrigerator or bathroom mirror for inspiration. You'll get there soon.

DON'T give your entire wardrobe to the Salvation Army just yet. It's cheaper to have things taken in than it is to replace them.

DO rest frequently and sleep longer if you feel like it. Indulge yourself in laziness from time to time.

DON'T allow yourself to get overtired. Fatigue is a dieter's enemy.

DO learn to reward yourself in ways that don't involve eating. Too often, we use food as a symbol of self-congratulation for a task well done.

DON'T feel as if you must avoid restaurants altogether. Remember that there's a Fast Lane Diet plan that tells you what and how to eat in those circumstances, too.

And, most of all, *do* pat yourself on the back for choosing the Fast Lane Diet!

No-Calorie and Low-Calorie Snacks for Fast-Laners

OK, so you've been good. You've stuck to the Fast Lane Diet plan of your choosing for two weeks, and you can already see results. But it's midafternoon at work, and you feel like chewing on something. Or it's midnight and you're yearning for a snack. Or friends have dropped by unexpectedly, and you're getting them a bite to eat, and you're afraid you'll stare at them rudely and drool if you don't eat, too—

It's all right. You don't have to deny yourself everything. There are plenty of treats you can indulge in without throwing your diet to the wind. Start with the obvious no-calorie ones— sugarless gum or hard candy, diet soda. Use your imagination to dress up a calorie-free drink:

- Stir a cup of herb tea with a fragrant cinnamon stick.
- Try an "exotic" diet soft-drink flavor—some brands come in chocolate!
- Rub a fresh slice of lime around the edge of a glass of spring water.

Bring some ceremony into the process: Serve your cup of decaffeinated coffee in your best china.

For almost anything else, calories count, so you'd better be prepared to count them. At the back of this book, you'll find a list of foods and the calories each contains per serving. Some of them won't surprise you. Here are some that will—each contains no more than 100 calories!

- 6 ounces of Chablis, served in a big glass with lots of ice
- 2 large, fresh, rosy peaches
- 1 dozen medium almonds
- 8 animal crackers
- 3 orange-flavored Kool Pops, or 1 orange Popsicle (Better yet: Freeze fresh fruit juice in an ice-cube tray.)
- 2 tablespoons of cream cheese (Roll each nibble around on your tongue.)
- 1 can light beer, almost any brand, ice-cold
- 5 teaspoons of honey (To prolong the pleasure, lick it off a finger.)
- 2 chocolate-covered graham crackers
- 10 raw oysters, smothered in hot sauce
- 2 empty sugar ice-cream cones (I mean *empty*.)
- 8 potato chips (the thin ones)
- 5 large prunes (Chew each sweet bite slowly.)

- 4 twisted thin pretzels
- $\frac{1}{20}$ of a 9-inch homemade lemon meringue pie (Immediately after eating your slice, take the rest of the pie to a neighbor's house.)
- 3 tablespoons of seedless raisins (brown or gold—it doesn't matter)
- 3 fresh purple plums
- 35 Goldfish cheddar crackers
- 2 cups of fresh strawberries
- 1 cup of red raspberries
- 1 enormous mango
- 3 tiny Tootsie Rolls
- 4 cups of popcorn (no butter—don't bother to salt the popcorn because salt won't stick well without fat anyway)
- 1 medium-sized homemade bran muffin, hot from the oven (again, no butter)
- 14 peppermint Life Savers
- 16 Spanish olives

Finally, for those moments when you feel extra special:

- 4 ounces of extra-dry champagne, in your best fluted glass

Find other favorite foods, check the packages for calories, and divvy up portions accordingly. You'll be amazed at what you can get away with.

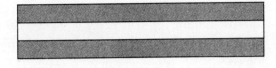

EPILOGUE

I've been putting this book together for some time now, and since I'm not a full-time writer, the creation of *The Fast Lane Diet* has *added* to my already frantic schedule.

But as I wrote and researched the book, I was living proof that the six Fast Lane Diets work. Throughout the past six and a half months, I have been on each of them. Each of the diets fitted into my specific fast lane needs at various times during the past year, and now it seems Tom and I have half of the people we know (and we know a lot of people) on the Fast Lane Diet Drink as part of their lifestyle. My 76-year-old mother uses it and loves it. And every once in a while I get a call from a friend or relative who's dreamed up a new recipe (some of which I've shared with you earlier in the book).

The Fast Lane Diet has helped to make me more confident. Confident that I can always stay at my ideal weight. Confident that I needn't change any of my demanding life in order to keep myself trim.

You should feel confident, too. You now have an alternative to time-absorbing, time-wasting, inefficient diets. You have the confidence that no matter how frantically busy you get, no matter how crowded your fast lane becomes, you will always be able to rely on the Fast Lane Diet to keep you on the straight and narrow whenever you need it.

No doubt you will make the Fast Lane Diet part of your fast lane life—for good.

APPENDIX:
Calorie Counter

(Asterisked foods are part of the Fast Lane Diet Program.)

Alcoholic beverages (*see* Distilled spirits;
Wine; Liqueurs)
Almonds*
  12 medium, *100*
  12 shelled unsalted, *105*
Apple*
  (2½ inch, 4 per pound), *61*
  (2¾ inch, 3 per pound), *80*
  (3¼ inch, 2 per pound), *123*
  1 medium Granny Smith, *61*
Applesauce, canned
  Del Monte, ½ cup, *100*
  Tillie Lewis, ½ cup, *60*
Apricots, 8 large dried halves, *80*
Artichoke*
  1 cold, cooked, dipped in 2 tablespoons
    sour cream, *125*
  braised Provençal style, *127*
Asparagus, 1 cup boiled, *29*
Avocado, 1 peeled and pitted, *300*

Bagel*
  ½ with 1 teaspoon butter or margarine,
    116
  ½ with no butter, *81*
  with lox and cream cheese, *374*
Banana*
  1 large, *119*
  1 medium, *103*
Bean burrito*, Taco Bell, *343*
Beans
  Great Northern, ½ cup, cooked, *100*
  green, cooked*
    1 cup, *31*
    ½ cup with almonds, 1 tablespoon,
      113
    ½ cup with Parmesan cheese, 1 table-
      spoon, *49*
  red kidney, cooked, 1 cup, *220*
Beef
  Arby's roast beef sandwich, *350**

Beef (continued)
Banquet beef pot pie (8 ounces), *400**
Burger King Whopper, Jr., *360**
flank steak, 4 ounces, broiled, with 1 tablespoon Worcestershire sauce, *224**
Gino's Sirloiner with cheese, *532*
Green Giant sloppy Joe with 1 bun, *270*
ground lean
¼ pound broiled, *186**
Cedric Adams casserole, 1 portion, *280**
Hardee's cheeseburger, *335*
McDonald's cheeseburger, *306*
Morton's beef enchilada (12-ounce pkg), *350**
Oriental with vegetables and rice (Stouffer's), *300**
White Castle cheeseburgers, 2, *370*
Beef jerky, 4 ¼-ounce sticks, *40**
Beef Stroganoff, Stouffer's frozen, *390**
Beef teriyaki, Stouffer's frozen 10-ounce pkg, *365**
Beer
light, 12 ounces, *100**
regular, 12 ounces, *150**
Beverages (see specific beverages)
Biscuit, Pillsbury buttermilk with 1 tablespoon low-calorie jam, *154**
Biscuits, Stella D'Oro egg, 2, *82**
Blueberries*
canned, Seabrook Farms ½ cup, *45*
fresh, ½ cup, *45*
fresh, 1 cup mixed with ¼ cup skim milk, *113*
Bologna, 1 piece, *90*
Bouillon, 1 cup hot instant*
Herb-Ox, *6*
Maggi, *6*
Wyler's, *6*
Boysenberries, S & W, ½ cup, *32*
Bread*
Dromedary date nut roll, ½-inch slice with 1 teaspoon cream cheese, *115*
English muffin, ½ with 1 tablespoon jam, *132*
French, 1 slice, *79*
hard roll, 1, *120*
Italian hard roll, no butter, *200*
melba toast (2 small slices), *70*

rye, 1 slice, *75*
Sara Lee cinnamon roll, 1, *146*
soft roll, 1, *90*
whole wheat, 1 slice, *60*
Breadsticks*
Stella D'Oro, *82*
sesame, 2, *106*
Broccoli, 1 cup cooked*
with butter, 1 tablespoon, *159*
with lemon juice, *63*
with Parmesan cheese, grated, 1 tablespoon, *89*
with sour cream, 2 tablespoons, *117*
Burrito, bean, Taco Bell, *343*
Butter, 1 tablespoon, *100*
Buttermilk, 1% fat, 8 ounces, *107*

Cabbage, 1 cup shredded, with 1 tablespoon diet mayonnaise and caraway seed, *57**
Cake
pound, 1 piece, *128*
homemade butter with boiled icing, ⅑ of 9-inch square, *401*
homemade butter with chocolate icing, ⅑ of 9-inch square, *453*
Candy
chocolate bar
Hershey's 1.2-ounce bar, *187*
Hershey's with almonds, 1.15 ounce, *180*
jelly beans, 1 ounce, *95**
licorice (Switzer), 1 ounce, *101**
Life Savers, 14 peppermint, *100**
M & M plain, 1½ ounces, *202*
3 Musketeers, 2 ounces, *254*
Raisinets, 1 ounce, *90**
Tootsie Rolls, 3 tiny, *100*
Canteloupe*, ½, *34*
½ topped with 1 tablespoon yogurt and chopped mint, *44*
Carrot*
boiled,
½ cup, *23*
1 cup, *45*
with 2 tablespoons cheddar cheese and 1 tablespoon chopped onion and dill, *81*
raw
½ cup sliced, *30*

1 cup, *95*
1 medium, *21*
  dipped in 2 tablespoons Dijon mus-
    tard, *51*
1 whole, *21*
2 whole, *42*
Celeri remoulade, *150*
Celery*
  2 stalks, *14*
  4 sticks stuffed with 3 tablespoons ched-
    dar cheese, *93*
Cereals
  1 cup cooked
    farina, *135*
    grits, *79*
    oatmeal, *160*
  1 cup ready-to-eat
    bran, *150*
    corn, *110*
    oat, *110*
    raisin bran, *200*
    rice, *110*
    wheat, *92*
    Wheat Chex, ⅔ cup, *110*
Champagne, 4 ounces dry, *100*
Cheese*
  American, 1 slice, *83*
  cream, 2 tablespoons, *100*
  Edam, 1 ounce, *100*
  farmer's, 1 ounce, *100*
  Gruyère, 1 ounce Swiss Knight or Bor-
    den's, *101*
  low-fat cottage
    ½ cup, *90*
    ½ cup served with sliced radish, *97*
  mozzarella, part skim milk, 1 ounce, *80*
  ricotta, ½ cup, *160*
Cheese blintz, 1 Golden with 2 table-
  spoons sour cream, *271*
Cheeseburger*
  Burger King, *360*
  Hardee's, *335*
  McDonald's, *306*
  White Castle, 2, *370*
Cherries*
  canned, ½ cup
  Del Monte light, *95*
  S & W, *50*
  fresh, sweet, 1 cup, *82*
Chick-peas, 1 cup, *720*

Chicken*
  à la king, Stouffer's, *330*
  breast
    broiled with skin removed, *154*
      seasoned with chopped celery and
        onion, *170*
  Dijon, *180*
  Chinese fried, average portion, *669*
  Church's fried, 1 piece, *315*
  La Choy frozen Chinese dinner, *354*
  moo goo gai pan, *248*
  pollo en salsa verde, average portion,
    244
  Weight Watchers chicken oriental, *240*
Chicken chow mein, average portion*
  Chun King, *330*
  with ½ cup each noodles and rice, *260*
Chicken liver*
  chopped, ½ cup, *116*
  sautéed, 4 ounces, *180*
Chicken Oriental, Weight Watchers, *240*
Chicken salad, *323*
Chicken with almonds, average portion,
  750
Chicken with Litchis, average portion, *250*
Chicken Yakitori, average portion, *250*
Chili*
  Dairy Queen chili dog, *330*
  Hormel beef without beans, 1 7½-ounce
    can, *344*
  Wendy's, *230*
Club soda, 8 ounces, *0*
Cocktails, alcoholic*
  bottled, 4 ounces
    black Russian, *368*
    grasshopper, *266*
    pīna colada, *240*
    tequila sunrise, *160*
  made using standard 1-ounce recipe
    rum Cola, *224*
    martini, *115*
    Irish coffee, *214*
    brandy Alexander, *225*
Cocoa
  commercial mixes, 6 ounces, *110*
  home recipe, 8 ounces, *242*
Cod, 4 ounces, broiled with butter, *200*
Coffee, 6 ounces, *2*
  flavored, 6 ounces, *60*
Coleslaw, average portion, *238*

Cookies*
  oatmeal, 1, *83*
  chocolate, 2 Oreo, *100*
  chocolate chip, 1, *53*
  Fig Newtons, 2, *120*
Corn, boiled
  kernels, 1 cup, *140*
  on the cob (1 5-inch ear), *70*
Corn chips, 1 ounce, *160*
Cornish hen, fat and skin removed, *162**
Crab
  deviled, 1 cup, *451*
  imperial, 1 cup, *451*
Crackers
  animal, 8, *100**
  Carr's table water
    large, *32*
    small, *15*
  cheese-flavored, 1 ounce, *136*
  Goldfish, 35 cheddar, *100**
  graham*
    2 chocolate-covered, *100*
    2 with 1 teaspoon grape jam on each,
      88
  oyster, 10, *33**
  Ritz*
    1 piece, *17*
    3 with 1 teaspoon cream cheese on
      each, *51*
  saltines, 1 piece, *12*
  sesame (Keebler)*
    2 with 1 teaspoon Brie cheese on each,
      54
  soda, 1 piece, *15*
  Triscuit*
    1 piece, *20*
    2 with 1 teaspoon peanut butter on
      each, *106*
  wheat thins*
    1 piece, *15*
    3 each spread with 1 teaspoon Snack-
      mate cheese spread, *78*
Cranberry-orange relish, 4 ounces, *202*
Cream
  half and half, 1 tablespoon, *19*
  heavy, 1 tablespoon, *52*
  light, 1 tablespoon, *25*
  medium, 1 tablespoon, *41*
Cream substitute
  Reddi-Whip, 1 teaspoon, *7*
  Sta-Whip, 1 teaspoon, *8*

Creamsicle, 1 orange, *80**
Croissant, 1 plain, *109**
Cucumber*
  1 whole, *29*
  Japanese, *48*
  salad, ½ cup, *48*

Dates, 1 cup pitted, *376*
Diet soda, 8 ounces, *1 or 2**
Distilled spirits, 1 ounce
  80 proof, *65*
  90 proof, *75*
  100 proof, *85*
  150 proof, *125*
Doughnut
  Hostess plain cinnamon or powdered
    sugar, *110**
  Jelly, 1, *175*
Egg
  1 hard-boiled, *81*
  omelet, 2-egg, made without butter and
    with sliced mushrooms, *172*
  scrambled, mixed with milk and cooked
    in fat, 1 cup, *381*
  stuffed, 1, *148*
Egg foo yung, average portion, *322**
Egg roll, *145**
Eggnog, dairy packed, 8 ounces, *302*
Eggplant Parmesan*
  Mrs. Paul's, *250*
  Weight Watchers, *280*
Enchilada*
  beef, 12-ounce frozen dinner, *479*
  cheese, 12-ounce frozen dinner, *459*
Espresso, *2*

Fast Lane Diet Drink*
  basic recipe, *220*
  Low-Lactose Milk, *140*
  No-Milk Diet Drink 1, *140*
  No-Milk Diet Drink 2, *129*
  variations, *275*
Fish*
  baked à la Fast Lane, *180*
  Coach Bud Grant's, *230*
  fillet, 4 ounces, *170*
    Arthur Treacher's, 2 pieces, *482*
    broiled without butter, 4 ounces, *125*
    Van de Kamp's 11-ounce pkg, *300*

white, 4 ounces, broiled, *170*
2 White Castle sandwiches, *384*
(*see also* specific kinds, e.g., Flounder)
Fish 'n' chips*
  Swanson Hungry Man (15¾-ounce pkg), *760*
  Swanson TV brand (10¼-ounce pkg), *450*
Fish stew, *200*
Flounder*
  baked with lemon and 1 tablespoon sliced almonds, 4 ounces, *288*
  broiled and seasoned with garlic and lemon, *170*
  Taste-o-Sea fried, *350*
Frankfurters, beef, 1 frank, *140*
Frankfurters and beans in tomato sauce, Heinz 8¾-ounce can, *399*
Fruit*
  1 ounce dried bits, *80*
  (*see also* specific fruits)
Fruit cocktail, canned, *75*
Fruit salad*
  canned, *80*

Gefilte fish, average portion with 1 tablespoon horseradish, *208*
Gelatin, 4-ounce serving*
  with low-fat topping, *90*
  diet, *10*
    with diet cherries, *100*
  Jell-O, *80*
Grapefruit, ½, *40*
Gravy, ¼ cup
  beef (Franco-American), *30*
  chicken (Durkee), *22*
    Weight Watchers, *10*
Guacamole, 1 tablespoon, *28*

Ham, cooked, 2 slices, *80*
Ham and cheese sandwich, Arby's, 5½ ounces, *380*
Hamburger (*see* Beef, ground)
Hollandaise sauce, ½ cup, *170*
Honey, 5 teaspoons, *100*
Horseradish, 1 ounce, *100*
Hot Dog with chili, Dairy Queen, *330*
(*see also* Frankfurters)
Huevo ranchero, 1 egg, *186*

Ice-cream cones, 2 empty, *100*

Juices, 6-ounce servings*
  apple, *80*
  Cranapple, *120*
  grape, *120*
  grapefruit, *70*
  orange, *85*
  prune, *13*
  tomato, *35*

Kool Aid, all flavors, *93*
Kool pops, 3 orange, *100*

Lamb chops, 2 broiled, *244*
Lasagne with meat sauce*
  Buitoni, *596*
  Stouffer's frozen 10½-ounce pkg, *385*
  Weight Watchers, with cheese, veal, and sauce, *350*
Lemon sorbetto, ½ cup, *70*
Lentils, ½ cup cooked, *107*
Linguini alle vongole (linguini with white clam sauce), 1½-cup serving, *350*
Liqueurs, 1 ounce, *100* average
Lobster Cantonese, average portion, *393*
Lobster
  meat only, 4 ounces, *108*
  Newburg, 4 ounces, *220*
Lox (*see* Salmon, smoked)

Macaroni and cheese, Swanson TV, *390*
Mango, 1 large, *100*
Margarine, 1 tablespoon
  diet, *50*
  imitation, *50*
  regular, *100*
Margarita, 8 ounces, *348*
Meatballs, average-sized, 2, *200*
Melba Toast, 5 rounds with 1 teaspoon low-fat cottage cheese on each, *107*
Milk, 8 ounces
  chocolate, *190*
    mixes, Carnation slender, *110*
  low-fat, *130*
    2 percent fat, *130*
  skim, *90*
  whole, *150*

Muffin, 1*
  blueberry, *120*
  bran, small, with no butter, *118*
  corn, *120*
  English, *130*
  raisin bran, *130*
Mushrooms*
  1 cup sautéed in bouillon or broiled, no fat, *20*
Mussels steamed in wine, *125**

Nachos, 4, *160**
Nectarine, 1 medium, *73**
Nondairy creamers, 1 teaspoon, *11*
Noodles*
  ½ cup cooked with 1 tablespoon Parmesan cheese
    1 tablespoon butter and ½ teaspoon capers, *190*
  ½ cup spinach or whole wheat
    with 2 tablespoons Parmesan cheese, parsley, celery, diced onion, ½ cup raw mushrooms, pepper, and garlic, *180*
  1 cup cooked with 1 tablespoon Parmesan cheese, *120*
  1 cup pasta shells, served cold with ½ cup low-fat cottage cheese, parsley, pepper, and garlic, *260*
Nuts, cashew, 10 medium, *75**

Oils, 1 tablespoon
  corn, *122*
  olive, *125*
  peanut, *128*
  safflower, *119*
  soybean, *128*
  sunflower, *120*
  vegetable, *120*
Olives, Spanish, 16, *100**
Omelet, with caviar, 1 egg, *180**
Orange*
  1 large, *73*
  1 medium, *64*
Orange roughy, 4 ounces, broiled, *129**
Oysters, 10 raw, *100**

Pancake, 1 4-inch, *62*
  with 1 tablespoon each butter and syrup, *205*
Pastrami, 1 slice, *45*
Peach
  1 medium, *38**
  2 large, *100**
  canned, ½ cup, *70*
  canned in heavy syrup, ½ cup, *95*
Pear, 1 Bosc, *101**
Peas, boiled, 1 cup, *115*
Pepper, green or red sweet*
  1 sliced, *11*
    dipped in 2 tablespoons low-fat yogurt, *43*
Pepperoni, 1 ounce, *145*
Pickle*
  genuine dill, *10*
  kosher dill, *2*
Pickle loaf, 1 piece, *70*
Pie, lemon meringue, ¹⁄₂₀ of 9-inch pie, *100**
Pineapple, 1 cup fresh, *80*
Pizza*
  Pizza Hut cheese pizza, 2 slices, *360*
  Stouffer's french bread, ½ package, *420*
  Weight Watchers sausage and cheese, *390*
Plums*
  3, purple, *100*
Popcorn*
  2 cups unbuttered, *50*
  4 cups, *100*
Popsicle, 1 twin, *70**
Pork
  chop, broiled, 4 ounces, lean only, *230*
  ham, 4 ounces, lean only, *246*
  loin roasted, 4 ounces, lean only, *288*
Potato
  1 baked in skin, *145**
    with 2 tablespoons low-fat cottage cheese and dill weed, *168**
    with ½ cup low-fat cottage cheese, chopped green pepper, and 2 tablespoons shredded cheddar cheese, broiled, *296**
    with 1 tablespoon butter, *245**
  1 medium boiled, topped with parsley and onion, *144**
  knish, *200**

mashed with milk and butter, 4 ounces, *107*
scalloped with cheese, 4 ounces, *118*
Potato chips, 8 thin, *100*
Pretzels*
 1 rod, *50*
 4 average twisted, thin, *100*
Prosciutto and melon, *120**
Prunes, 5 large, *100**

Radish*
 4 sliced, *7*
Raisins, 3 tablespoons, *100**
Raspberries*
 fresh
  black, 1 cup, *98*
  red, 1 cup, *70*
  with ricotta cheese, 1 teaspoon, *100*
 frozen, Bird's Eye, ½ cup, *120*
Ravioli
 beef, 7½ ounces, *230*
 cheese, 7½ ounces, *260*
 Buitoni 15-ounce can, *408*
Red snapper, 4 ounces, broiled, *105**
Rice*
 brown, ½ cup cooked, *110*
 white, ½ cup cooked, *100*

Salad, 1 cup*
 green, without dressing, *10*
 green, with 2 tablespoons low-calorie Italian dressing, *60*
 green onion and celery, 1 sliced orange, topped with 1 tablespoon sliced almonds and 2 tablespoons low-calorie Italian dressing, *248*
 spinach leaves, mushrooms, 1 tablespoon sunflower seeds, 1 tablespoon raisins and 2 tablespoons low-calorie Italian dressing, *189*
 taco, without sour cream or guacamole, *250**
 tomato, sliced, and radish, *37*
Salad Bar*
 with lettuce, bean sprouts, cucumber, radishes, green peppers, 1 table-spoon grated cheese, and 1 teaspoon bacon bits, with 1 tablespoon diet dressing, *180*
 with mixed greens, cucumber, radishes, 1 tablespoon shredded cheese, and 1 tablespoon diet dressing, *125*
Salad dressing, 1 tablespoon*
 Bleu cheese, *70*
 Caesar, *70*
 diet, *25*
 French, *56*
 French creamy, *62*
 Italian, *50*
 Italian creamy, *70*
 Russian creamy, *80*
Salad Niçoise, *305**
Salami
 1 ounce, *327*
 1 slice, *50*
Salmon, simple (for a crowd), *1,924**
 smoked, 4 ounces, *200**
Sandwiches, average-size
 corned beef, *450*
 pastrami, *550*
 roast beef, *500*
 tuna fish salad, *350*
Sashimi, 4 ounces, assorted, *100**
Sauce, ½ cup
 béarnaise, *176*
 Bordelaise, *48*
 cheese, *160*
 hollandaise, *170*
 spaghetti, canned, meatless, *120*
Sausage
 breakfast, 1 link, *78*
 Italian, 3-ounce link, *271*
Scallops*
 4 ounces, broiled, *127*
 with vegetables on white rice, *270*
Scones, 1, *188*
Scrapple, 1 ounce, *45*
Seltzer, *0*
Sherbet*
 1 cup, *260*
 Baskin-Robbins daiquiri ice, 1 scoop, *99*
 Baskin-Robbins orange, 1 scoop, *84*
 rainbow, 1 scoop, *100*
Sherry, 4 ounces
 cream, *175*
 dry, *140*

Shrimp*
  8 ounces, peeled, sautéed in lime juice
    and ½ teaspoon oil, *240*
  Arthur Treacher's, *380*
Shrimp balls, *286*
Shrimp chow mein, Chun King, *360**
Shrimp cocktail, 4-ounce jar, Sau-Sea, *112**
Shrimp toast, *162*
Sloppy Joe, Green Giant boil-in-bag, with
    1 hamburger bun, *270**
Soda, 8 ounces
  Birch beer, *110*
  Bitter lemon, *128*
  Cherry, *122*
  Coca-Cola, *96*
  diet, *1 or 2**
  Dr. Brown's Cel-Ray tonic, *89**
  Dr. Brown's cream soda, *127**
  ginger ale, *85*
  Pepsi Cola, *104*
  quinine water, *88*
  root beer, *110*
  7-Up, *97*
  Sprite, *95*
Soufflé
  Stouffer's cheese, *241*
  Stouffer's corn, *154*
Soup, 1 cup*
  beef consommé, *10*
  beef with vegetables, *61*
  beef, *286*
  borscht, *75*
  chicken broth with egg (stracciatella),
    *125**
  chicken broth with escarole, *138*
  chicken with vegetables, *80*
  Chinese crab combination, *150*
  Chinese pork and vegetable, *187*
  clam chowder
    Manhattan, *74*
      with ¼-ounce canned clams plus 1
        cup skim milk, *274*
    New England, *140*
  egg drop, average portion, *89*
  cream of carrot (without the cream, à la
    Fast Lane), *65**
  cream of chicken, Lipton Cup-a-Soup,
    80
  gazpacho, average portion, *192*
  hot and sour, average portion, *275*
  lentil, 1 cup canned, *150*

miso
  with bean curd, *79*
  with fish balls, *142*
mushrooms in broth, *80*
quick crab, *120**
Santé potage, *150**
sesame chicken, average portion, *301*
split pea with ham, *180*
stracciatella, *49**
vichyssoise, low-calorie, *107**
Soy sauce, 1 teaspoon, *7*
Spaghetti*
  Buitoni, with meatballs, 15-ounce can,
    456
  with cream and Parmesan cheese (alla
    panna e parmigiano), 1½-cup serv-
    ing, *315*
  with tomato sauce (in salsa al pomodoro
    romano), 1½- to 2-cup serving, *375-
    400*
  Stouffer's, 1 package Lean Cuisine por-
    tion with meatballs, *300*
Spam, 1 ounce, *85*
Spinach*
  1 cup cooked, *41*
    mixed with 1 tablespoon yogurt and
      seasoned with garlic, *46*
  raw, 1 cup chopped, *14*
Squash, acorn, ½ baked with 1 teaspoon
    butter or margarine, *35**
Steak, broiled, lean only, *254**
Strawberries*
  fresh, 1 cup, *55*
    with 2 tablespoons low-fat yogurt, *73*
  frozen, Bird's Eye, ½ cup, *90*
Sukiyaki, Chun King stir fry, ⅓ pkg, *100**
Sushi, tekka maki, *400**
Sweet and sour carp, average portion, *450**
Sweet rolls, cinnamon, average-size, *100**
Swordfish, broiled, 4 ounces, *185**

Taco*
  beef, 2 Taco Bell, *372*
  chicken, *160*
  shrimp, *145*
Tea*
  6 ounces, *1*
  iced, mix, with sugar and lemon, 6
    ounces, *60*

Tomato*
baked with 1 tablespoon breadcrumbs, *75*
1 broiled with 1 tablespoon Parmesan cheese, oregano, and garlic powder, *55*
sliced with onion, oil, and vinegar, *50*
Tortilla chips*
nacho cheese flavored,
4, dipped in salsa, *40*
1 ounce, *140*
Tuna*
noodle casserole, Stouffer's, *400*
open-face rolls, *170**
salad, with 6½-ounce can tuna fish packed in water, 1 hard-boiled egg, 1 tablespoon diet mayonnaise, celery, onion, garlic, and lemon juice, *360*
Turkey, 4 ounces*
roast
dark meat, *230*
light meat, *200*
smoked, 1 slice with dill spear, *37*

Veal*
parmigiana, Green Giant 7-ounce pkg, *310*
plain, sautéed in butter, 4 ounces, *245*
Vegetables, mixed cooked, 1 cup, *130**

Watermelon, 1 cup, diced, *42**
Wine*
dry red, 4 ounces, *96*
dry white, 4 ounces, *90*

Yogurt*
frozen, Danny Yogurt-on-a-Stick, uncoated, 1, *65*
plain, Sweet 'n' Low, 1 8-ounce container, *90*

Zucchini, 1 sliced, *9**